RESCUING PROVIDENCE AND RESCUE 1 RESPONDING

MICHAEL MORSE

A POST HILL PRESS BOOK

ISBN (trade paperback): 978-1-61868-799-9

RESCUING PROVIDENCE AND RESCUE 1 RESPONDING
© 2016 by Michael Morse
All Rights Reserved

Cover Design by Christian Bentulan

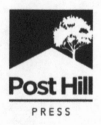

Post Hill Press
275 Madison Avenue, 14th Floor
New York, NY 10016
http://posthillpress.com

RESCUING

PROVIDENCE

"We few. We happy few. We band of brothers."

—*King Henry V*

A fortunate man has three great loves in his life. Mine all came at once. For Cheryl, Danielle, and Brittany.

PROLOGUE

0230 hrs

"Rescue 1, are you available?"

"Roger, what have you got?"

"Respond to Providence College for a student who has fallen off of a roof."

"Rescue 1, on the way."

We were worn out, finishing a thirty-eight. Lori hit the lights and siren and changed direction, driving toward the incident.

It only took a minute to get there. The campus was quiet, most of the kids slept or crammed for finals. Lifeless soccer fields, empty administration buildings and classrooms led us toward the brick seven story dormitory. Twenty-five years ago ten girls jumped to their deaths from one of the dorms here, trying to escape a fire that started when some festive decorations lining the walls ignited. They couldn't wait for the ladders that would have rescued them, the flames too hot and smoke too thick. Some crashed to the ground in front of their rescuers, seconds away from salvation. It was the worst day in the history of the Providence Fire Department. We have had more than our share of bad days.

A security guard directed us up a hill to the base of St. Joseph's Hall. Another guard had a student in his grasp, his anguish evident as he weakly fought to get free, his guttural wails echoing off of the buildings.

At the top of the hill and the base of the building, lying in a crumbled heap was our victim. I got out of the rescue and walked closer, hoping beyond hope that this was some bizarre prank. It wasn't.

I am a firefighter. People look to me when they need help. The crumbled heap was a kid named John. He looked at me through eyes that were popped from their sockets yet miraculously still focused on my own. He tried to speak; blood and teeth flowed from his mouth rather than words.

"It's bad," I said to Lori as she wheeled the stretcher close. With help from Engine 12 who had been called to assist we immobilized our patient then loaded him into the truck and headed for the trauma room at Rhode Island Hospital, the area's only Level 1 trauma center. John fought for life all the way. His broken bones were hinged in multiple places, as he moved his shoulders and hips the limbs went in opposite directions. The hat he wore, a light brown wool cap with earflaps that tie if you want finally fell from his head onto the blood-splattered floor of the rescue. I remembered hats like from my childhood, when mothers and grandmothers would bundle their kids up before sending them into the cold. They have regained their popularity with older kids; it's funny how things come and go. I picked it up and placed it on his chest, the only part of his body that didn't appear outwardly broken. Inside, his vital organs were a scrambled mess. He somehow gathered the strength to grasp my wrist as I tried to keep him from moving. I was amazed both by the power still exuding from his broken body and the emotional response his desperate gesture had on me. The mangled mass of flesh and bone became more to me than I had intended, my quest to distance myself from the emotional carnage that lay ahead destroyed. His grip on my arm went directly to my heart, breaking once we become more intimate. I wondered to myself, who am I to be present and in charge as this drama unfolds? I'm just a regular guy who a few years ago couldn't manage his own life, never mind leading a team of firefighters in this grim effort.

I put aside my self-doubt and marched on, no time for indecision when a life hung in the balance. The responsibility is sometimes overwhelming, but worrying about it doesn't help anybody.

I'm certain the look on the faces of Lori and the guys from Engine 12 mirrored my own. I saw horror and pity mixed with revulsion in their expressions as we worked. We did all we could, started IV's, gave oxygen and tried to comfort our patient while we endured what for some of was is the longest ride of our career.

An hour after we handed what was left of John over to the emergency room staff I sat on the floor outside the trauma room, state report on my knees, the empty spaces waiting to be filled. My hand held a pen that I couldn't get going. The guys from Engine 12 were in the barn waiting for the next alarm. Lori was with the triage nurses who were busy with the kid who had witnessed his best friend fall eighty feet from the slippery dorm roof.

The boys had finished cramming for their exams and were sneaking onto the roof for a smoke. A window in a janitor's closet provided access to the roof if you were careful. This wasn't the first time the window was used. A beautiful view of the city was the reward for those daring enough to make the trip. The first boy made it onto the roof then waited for John. Something happened; he slipped and started sliding down the roof toward the edge. It happened fast. John's friend witnessed him go over, he then somehow made it back through the window, out of the closet and down the stairs to the first floor. He ran out the front door of the dorm to see if he could help. He was the first to see the result of an eighty-foot fall onto frozen ground. John was critically injured, his friend's life forever changed by what he saw. I can only hope he gets the help he needs and doesn't push it away as guys his age are prone to do.

From the corner of my eye, a priest appeared at the end of the long corridor we call "trauma alley." The hospital's six trauma rooms line the narrow hallway, filled with the most advanced medical equipment available. At a moments notice these rooms can be filled with trauma teams consisting of doctors, nurses, respitory experts and support staff. Now, most were empty. One of the rooms showed signs of activity; a lone janitor mopping buckets of blood from the floor. John had been taken upstairs to surgery.

Two people joined the priest and they made their way toward me under the bright fluorescent lights up trauma alley. They were my age, dressed is sweatshirts and sweatpants, things found at a moments notice, no coats. They clung to each other, the man holding the woman up, supporting her as they made the long walk toward an uncertain future that seemed so bright when the fell asleep hours before, now shrouded with uncertainty and fear. I knew why they were here and the bad news that awaited them, hoping beyond hope that everything would be as it was they struggled past me. I cowardly looked down at my empty report and pretended to write, not wanting to see up close the effects of this tragedy any more that night.

They were a close, religious family from a nearby Massachusetts town, Mom, Dad and three kids. They sent their son to a Catholic college hoping he would be safe. They walked past, never knowing it was me who peeled their son off of the curb at the bottom of his dorm and held him together through the ride to the hospital. I know he would have died on the pavement if not for our intervention. I get some satisfaction knowing his parents will have the opportunity to hold their child once more while life flows through his veins. Whether that will be enough in the hard years to come I will never know. I don't think he will make it much longer.

Somehow I finished the report, helped Lori clean the rescue and limped back to the station. All quiet there. The engine and ladder company didn't turn a wheel all night. In my office a stack of reports waited to be logged into the computer. Thirteen runs, I had three hours to go. I hadn't slept in days; was exhausted, depressed and dirty. Too tired to shower or log the reports into the computer system, I collapsed onto my bunk. Mercifully I slept until my relief woke me at seven. After an hour doing reports I was on my way home. I turned on the radio, hoping to hear some music and clear my head. It was the top of the hour; my favorite station does a five-minute news segment at this time on weekdays. The story of the student who fell from the seventh floor of his dorm led the news. He was reportedly still in critical condition. I listened to the details, amazed at how cold and generic the information sounded when recounted by somebody who was just reading the news. My mind was still full of every minute detail, the smell of blood mixed with diesel fumes from the truck's exhaust, similar to charred meat cooking on a propane grill, tension from the rescuers, horror from the witnesses and the victim's pain all mixed together forming a cloud of desperation that can be felt only by those who were there. You could tell the story a hundred times and the people hearing the story will never feel it, can never appreciate what goes on. Only those unfortunate souls who live through such experiences bear the full weight of the memories.

PART I

ONE

Minutes before ruining the morning tranquility I disabled my alarm clock, giving me a few more precious moments of peace. Beside me, my wife was sleeping, softly breathing. I'd been awake since four, lying in the dark, alone with my thoughts. I couldn't get the events from last week out of my mind. I left the city exhausted, physically and emotionally drained after working seventy-two hours in four days. I've had a few days off; it was time to get back to work. I'd have preferred to lie there forever, warm, safe and happy. I couldn't. In an hour, it will be time to go.

I had managed to forget almost everything about last week, forcing the memories deep into my subconscious mind where I hoped they stay forever. Some things refuse to stay buried. The kid who fell off the roof has to make room as another painful image crosses my mind. Lying safely in my bed I let it in, closed my eyes and drifted back to Broad Street.

I remembered a good-looking kid dying, a bullet hole in the middle of his chest and another in his abdomen. He was fifteen. The bravado that helped him survive on the streets left him, snuffed out like the spark of life that faded in front of me.

I don't like lying to people who I know will be dead in minutes. It doesn't seem fair. It's hypnotic in the back of a rescue when the

11

fight for life is lost and resignation appears in the victim's face. I tell them to hang on, keep fighting, but they know the truth. I can see it in their eyes. The last thing they see before leaving this earth forever is me. Going back to work to do it again is something I dread.

My old station wagon waited for me in the driveway, windows covered with frost. Leaving my family inside the house, I got in and started her up. Having no time for the defroster to do the job, I drove while peering out of the tiny porthole I made by scraping the windshield. The world seems a small place when viewed from a moving vehicle through a tiny hole. I had a fifteen-minute ride to the station; the view should have cleared by then.

The first traces of dawn touched the sky as I left the suburbs and headed toward the city. Some of the homes lining my street showed signs of life as I passed. Lights in the little upstairs windows appeared, soon to be frosted with steam from the shower. My windshield cleared as I navigated the turns in the road that hugs upper Narragansett Bay. To my left sat homes of affluent families, their lawns glistening with frost. People are drawn to the area, seduced by the magnificent view. To my right, fog rolled in with the sunrise creating a mystical illusion as reds and orange from the rising sun mixed with the cool blue of the water and the fog's whiteness. I've heard that seals swim in these waters though I have never seen one here. Every day that I travel this road I look, thinking today will be the day. Silhouettes of rocks that form the breakwater appeared through the mist; I knew that the seals were just beyond.

Ten minutes from my home, about a mile past the water view I entered another world. Providence's skyline appeared on the horizon creating an impressive backdrop in the distance. Homes are mixed with businesses on the main street, the side streets are lined with tenement houses we call 'triple deckers.' When I started my career with the fire department, a lot of these houses were vacant.

Elderly people hanging on to memories of more prosperous times lived in some of the old homes, poor people with nowhere else to go filled a few.

The area has benefited from an improving economy. One by one the homes are being repaired. The houses on these streets once again are filled with people, and a diverse community has appeared. Spanish and English are heard, sometimes a mixture of the two. What crime exists is underground and mostly out of sight. Families live here in relative safety, optimism replacing despair so prevalent years ago.

The Port of Providence dominates the waterfront. Oil tankers make their way from the Atlantic down the Providence River to the tank farms. Metal recycling and other industry fill the shoreline. It is a popular dumping ground for stolen cars. An occasional body will be discovered here as well. Last Christmas morning I responded to the area for a "man down." I found a twenty-year old with a bullet in his head. His lifeless eyes stared blankly, not seeing the bleak landscape, his skin the same gray as the frozen pavement he died upon. The security guard that found the body was shaking, maybe from the cold, maybe not. We looked at the corpse for a while, our breaths more rapid than usual, frozen mist as we exhaled the only movement on the deserted street. My radio cracked and interrupted the spell.

"Rescue 1, will the police be needed?" came the dispatchers monotone through the mike clipped to my coat.

"Roger, this is a crime scene with a DOA."

"Message received, police are on the way."

"Rescue 1 in service, and Merry Christmas."

I put the mike back into its clip, got in the rescue and waited for the police as the security guard stood over the body, lost in his own thoughts, my hopes for a quiet Christmas morning with my second family shattered.

The dead guy was a street hustler, fond of preying on gay men, charging them for his favors then sometimes beating and robbing them. The police are still sorting out the circumstances surrounding his murder. My guess is he robbed the wrong guy and ended up on the wrong end of the gun that put a hole in his head.

A few blocks from the fire station, high school students wait for the bus by the side of the road. I enjoy my morning and the peace it brings but I know the kids do not. It seems like yesterday that I was in their place, dreading the early mornings and wondering why school started so early. Though we live in a different world and time, we share the same hopes and dreams. Adolescent frustration feels the same now as it did then, whether growing up in the suburbs in the seventies or in the city today.

I saw flashing lights in front of my destination. Rescue 1 was on the ramp. I hoped that it was coming back from a run, not going out. Seeing the relief on Vinny's face as I pulled in told me all I needed to know; they were going. Another day had begun.

Wednesday, 0657 hrs. (6:57 a.m.)

"The truck's all set," said Vinny.

"How was your week?" I asked.

"What do you mean?" he said.

Vinny, the Captain of Rescue 1 is a fifteen-year veteran. I've never gotten a strait answer from him but always try. I'm sure that he worked a lot of overtime this week. He never complains, just keeps plugging along. He is my age, forty-two, but looked much older.

"Where are we going?" I asked him.

"50 Prairie Avenue for a terrible tragedy, everybody's waiting for you, hurry," he responded in a deadpan voice.

I knew that Vinny was exhausted as I was when he relieved me four days ago. He opened the door, got out, and I got in. He handed me the portable radio. The torch has been passed.

Mike was behind the wheel, grinning.

"Rescue 1, are you responding?" boomed the radio.

"Rescue 1 on the way," I said into the mike.

"Rescue 1 and Engine 3 responding at 0657 hours."

The cab of the rescue, a 2003 Ford F-350 diesel powered workhorse looked exactly the same as it did four days ago. The "wharf rat" sat on the dash, ever vigilant. He has been in the same spot for years, his plastic tail stuffed into a crack in the plastic. If rats could talk, the stories they could tell.

I adjusted my seat. Vinny likes to move the seat forward and recline the back as far as it will go. I prefer to sit as strait as possible. Lingering body odor wafted from the back, invading our space. It smelled like day old shit, and probably was. A lot of our patients live on the street and are more worried about survival than hygiene. Considering the amount of work the truck does it is remarkably well kept; a testament to the work ethic of the people assigned here.

A lot happens in this truck. Lives are lost, futures altered, hope abandoned and then reborn. Time relentlessly moves forward, impervious that some of the people who enter Rescue 1 are changed forever. We go into peoples homes and take them away, sometimes for months while they recuperate from whatever ails them. If they are fortunate they return home to find that for them, time stopped while the rest of the world kept moving. They tear off the calendar's pages, stopping when they reach the present day. Some never return, are either put in the grave or moved to a nursing facility. Family members are reminded how fragile our existence and tenuous our grasp on life is when they clean out their loved ones homes and see evidence of the final days. Newspapers, phone messages and mail, sometimes months old bear the date of the accident or illness serving as a grim reminder of the day when for them, time stood still.

I didn't expect a 'terrible tragedy' at our destination. Years of working with Vinny have made me aware of his ways. If this truly were a life-threatening emergency, he wouldn't have waited for me. Between true emergencies we transport a lot of non-emergency patients. Some people's idea of an emergency needing a fire department response differs from others.

Sirens filled the morning air, flashing lights mixed with the colors of the rising sun, bouncing off buildings and reflecting off glass as we made our way to our patient through the back streets and light early morning traffic. Fifty Prairie Avenue is a Hi-Rise with six floors and about 200 apartments. Most of the folks living there are elderly people on fixed incomes.

"How were your days off?" I asked Mike. He is relatively new to the job, three years, but has an unusual knack for the work we do.

"Henry's birthday party was a huge success," he said.

"Was the house ready in time?"

"Sixty people were there and not a single complaint."

"How did Amy handle it?"

"She did all right, got a little tired toward the end though. I'm glad Sammy slept through the whole thing. He's more work at a month old than Henry is at two years."

We rode to our destination in comfortable silence. I see more of Mike than I do my wife.

Mike steered the rescue into the parking lot of the hi-rise and parked behind Engine 3. We got the stretcher from the back of the rig and headed for the elevator. A minute later we were inside our patient's apartment. She was an elderly woman, sitting in her well-kept kitchen on a chair, shaking. Spices and pans sat neatly on the kitchen counter waiting to be put into use. Pictures of her smiling grandchildren were held by magnets on front of an old

Westinghouse refrigerator, cheering up the old appliance. Blood spattered the kitchen floor. She was conscious and alert, with some swelling around her eyes and a bloody nose.

"What happened?" I asked, crouching to her eye level.

"I was walking into the kitchen and fell flat on my face," she responded.

"Did you feel dizzy and faint or just trip?"

"My feet got all tangled up and I fell flat on my face!"

We put a cervical collar around her neck and had her lay flat on a long backboard, keeping her neck and back aligned, and put her on our stretcher. I had her pinch her nose and gave her a towel to control the bleeding. Mike assessed the woman's vital signs and we made our way to the elevator to the rescue.

The crew of Engine 3 assisted us as we loaded the patient into the truck. I noticed that Donna was not with them. She was helping load a motor vehicle accident victim into the rescue a few weeks ago. While lifting the stretcher into the back of the truck, she heard and felt a "pop" in her sternum area. Further tests indicated the presence of a growth behind the breastbone. She is a great kid, one of the few women on the department and very well liked throughout the job. We deal with sick people all day long with detached efficiency, but when it's one of us, the reality of our vulnerability hits home. This job has a way of making you feel invincible; untouched by the sickness and suffering we surround ourselves with daily. It seems inconceivable that one of our own may have succumbed to something only "other" people have to deal with. I hope she is all right.

"Blood pressure 124/78, pulse 80 and her glucose level is 124." It looks like you're going to live forever with those vitals," Mike said to the woman before leaving the back of the truck to drive. I stayed in the back with the patient. She didn't seem the talkative type so I respected her wishes as we made the two-minute ride in silence. The radio was tuned to the local rock station, Led Zeppelin blending perfectly with the siren providing a nice background for our short journey.

The hospital is in the middle of a major expansion and the temporary rescue entrance is right next to the construction site. I can only imagine what the patients think as we wheel them past the work crew. I don't notice the chaos anymore.

Rhode Island Hospital is Southern New England's designated level 1 Trauma Center. They have been treating people on the grounds since 1863. It serves as the major teaching hospital for Brown University's Medical School. Over six thousand people work there. In 2004, 114,888 patients were seen in the emergency room making it one of the busiest in the country.

The sweet smell of fresh vomit mingled with antiseptic greeted us. Ron, today's triage R.N. was at the desk. Rhode Island is a small place, and everybody seems connected somehow. My brother and Ron were members of the 1207th transportation unit of the Rhode Island National Guard until Ron retired. With the war in Iraq raging with no end in sight we have a lot to talk about. The 1207th was deployed last January. Ron had gotten out by that time but still inquires about his old Army friends. No time for small talk today, the ER is too busy. I gave a detailed description of my patient's chief complaint, medical history, prescriptions taken and allergies. Ron signed the State report and the patient belonged to him.

On the way out of the ER I stopped and talked to Domingo, one of the security guards. Emergency rooms in the city can be a wild place. RIH is no different. Six guards are always on duty. They all look competent, are large and act professionally.

"Mike! You doin ok this morning?"

"Fine Domingo, how's your daughter?" I asked.

"Five years old and the smartest one in her school. You know that she goin to be president one day?"

"I hope she runs as a Republican."

"Don even say that," Domingo replied in mock outrage, "When she is president we be eatin losster every day!" He says lobster without the "B", so it sounds funny. Every time he says it I laugh out loud.

"A Losster in every pot!" I said, and walked back to the truck. Mike was waiting, truck cleaned, the cervical collar restocked and everything ready to go.

TWO

The City of Providence is home to about 180,000 people. During the workweek that number swells to 350,000. On nights and weekends thousands more flood downtown for the clubs, theaters and other activities. The city's Fire Department consists of five hundred members manning fifteen engine companies, eight ladder trucks and five rescues. Three battalion chiefs, fire prevention, training, communications, arson investigators and administrative chiefs round out the department. We are the second oldest paid fire department in the country, Cincinnati being first. For over 150 years we have kept the city safe. Fourteen fire stations strategically placed throughout the city enable us to respond to most emergencies within minutes.

Four different platoons ensure twenty-four hour, seven-day coverage at the least cost to the city. We work two ten-hour days followed by two fourteen-hour nights, forty-eight hours a week. When overtime is available we work between shifts. Two groups work every day with the other two off. The schedule takes some getting used to, but once adjustments are made, the hours work out well. Working first, second and third shift eventually take a toll, but it is manageable.

Mike stopped the truck in front of the Dunkin Donut's shop on Eddy Street and asked, "What do you want, I'm buying?"

"Large coffee, just milk. Thanks"

"You coming in?"

"Not this time."

"Alright, see you in a few."

He headed into the donut shop and I took my cell phone out of my top pocket and called Cheryl. I had only left home a little while ago, but like to call from work to say good morning. For fourteen of our twenty years together I've been a firefighter. The long hours make it hard to keep a relationship fresh, but we do a pretty good job of it. She answered after a few rings. I could tell by the husky tone of her voice I had called too early.

"Hey babe, did I wake you up?" I asked.

"No, I was sleeping anyway," she answered. Still fresh.

"Sorry. I'm probably working tonight, there's an opening at Rescue 3."

"Call me later."

"Love you, bye."

"Love you too."

I clicked off the phone as Mike walked back to the rescue, his hands each held a large coffee and a bag dangled between his teeth. The bag probably held a breakfast croissant with cheese and sausage. I don't know where he puts it. He doesn't carry an ounce of extra fat on his five foot ten inch frame. He was wearing the trial uniform shirt. The traditional uniform is a light blue collared shirt with dark blue work pants. A white, yellow, black and red patch with the words "Providence Fire Department" around the sides and the slogan "In omnia paratus" in the middle adorns the left sleeve. "In Omnia Paratis", the slogan of the Providence Fire Department, is a Latin slogan meaning, 'In All Things, Prepared.' A black belt and black shoes complete the uniform. We don't wear a badge because we don't want to be confused with the police. A few members have been issued black polo shirts to wear on a trial basis. Mike is wearing one today.

"That shirt looks stupid," I said.

"Oh man, what are you talking about, this is the future."

"Then the future looks stupid too. Thanks for the coffee, I'll get you later."

The new shirts are a hit with most of the guys. Call me old-fashioned, but I prefer the more formal look of a button down collar. A polo shirt belongs on the golf course.

I keyed the mike on the truck radio. "Rescue 1 is in service." We were at the mercy of the dispatchers. Before we made it back to the station, the truck radio came to life.

0840 hrs. (8:40 a.m.)

"Rescue 1 and Engine 9, a still alarm." cracked the radio.

When somebody picks up the phone and calls the fire department it is called a still alarm. A box alarm means a mechanized alarm has been activated, a still box usually indicates there is a fire.

"Rescue 1 and Engine 9, respond to the corner of Wickenden and Benefit Streets in a silver Saab for a possible overdose."

"Rescue 1 on the way," I said into the mike.

We headed toward the East Side, about four miles from Allen's Avenue. Rescue 5 from the North Main Street station should have been first due there but they must have been on another call. When one rescue is busy, the next closest one is called. Sometimes things get crazy and the closest rescue is three towns away.

The East Side of Providence has a distinct personality, different from the rest of the city in a lot of ways; money, and lots of it being the biggest. Brown University dominates the area. Many of the historic homes that line the residential streets are owned by the university and rented to students, professors and support staff.

While contributing greatly to the city's cultural and academic status, the college contributes next to nothing to the tax base.

We drove over the Point Street Bridge toward Wickenden Street. Engine 9 was already there, no silver Saab in sight. The officer in charge of Engine 9 signaled with a shrug of his shoulders, the universal communication. This happens a lot. Somebody takes too many drugs, overdoses and becomes unresponsive, their friends panic and call for help, then realize the trouble they have brought upon themselves and drive away, hoping the problem goes away. Sometimes it does, sometimes not. I have found numerous addicts dead where their friends left them.

I informed the dispatchers through a radio transmission, "Rescue 1 to fire alarm, nobody on scene at Brook and Wickenden, we're going to look around the area."

We drove up Wickenden, the street was full of people even at this early hour. Antique shops displayed their wares in store windows, restaurants were full with the breakfast crowd and traffic had picked up. A homeless man stood at the end of a highway off ramp holding a sign saying "Homeless Vietnam Vet." Some cars stopped and put something in the can he held. A few hours later he cashed his earnings in at a local package store. Later still one of the city's rescues responded to the area to help a man found lying in the street. They found the "Homeless Vietnam Vet" drunk and hostile. He was taken to an Emergency Room for treatment.

The air was crisp; early spring in New England doesn't offer much relief from winters' grasp, yet after months of bitter cold, a forty-five degree day on a sun filled morning fills the most jaded pessimist with hopes of warmth. A brave few drank their coffee while sitting at sidewalk tables the coffee shops provide, warming their hands with steam rising from their cups. As the temperature rose, the tables filled.

On the way back to the station I spotted a silver Saab stopped in an intersection. The passenger seat occupant was kneeling backwards on the seat leaning into the back. His pants had drooped, exposing half of his ass.

"Mike, look, someone is smiling at you!" I said, pointing at the car. He spotted the buttocks.

Grinning, he said, "I thought the moon was gone for the day."

The car pulled behind us, horn blaring as we made our way onto the Point Street Bridge. I brought the radio to life.

"Rescue 1 to fire alarm, we have the overdose, have Engine 9 meet us at Point and Richmond.

"Engine 9 received."

The car followed us over the bridge and into a parking lot at Point and Richmond. I got out and walked to the car. I saw a man leaning over the front seat, his pants worn gangsta' style has slipped to his knees. He was trying to help a young girl in the back. She was barely breathing, her skin ashen.

"What's going on?" I asked the driver. I put on some rubber gloves, the pale purple latex free material stretching over my hands, giving me minimal protection should I be exposed to bodily fluids. Slowly, the rest of the crew followed suit.

"I don't know, she just stopped breathing," he responded.

"Heroin?"

"Yeah."

The man was reluctant to admit to illegal drug use, but saw the seriousness of the situation. The girl in the back of the car was in respiratory distress. She had overdosed, and would die in minutes without intervention. With help from the three members of Engine 9 we pulled the unconscious girl from the rear of the Saab and into the back of the rescue. As soon as we were done, I saw the silver Saab speed away.

I knew that the other firefighters had been through this ritual numerous times, and I imagine the victim has as well. Without a word from me, the girl is placed on high flow oxygen, a firefighter assisting ventilations with a device called a bag-valve mask. Her vital signs were assessed and an IV was started. While the crew did their thing, I drew up some Narcan, which counteracts the effects of narcotics. It is our most utilized drug.

"Pulsox eighty-two %, Blood pressure 60/40, respiration's 6, she's in respiratory arrest," said Mike. The syringe was ready.

"Watch out," I said to the guys. Sometimes the patient vomits violently when they regain consciousness. Narcan gives instant withdrawal.

I pinched off the line, pushed the drug then flushed. The medication was on the way. The five of us sat back and waited Slowly her color returned and she began breathing on her own.

"You are in a rescue with the fire department," I told her as she woke up. Her look of confusion turned into anger as she realized what was going on.

"What happened, where are my friends?" she asked.

Mark, one of the firefighters from Engine 9 let her have it.

"You and your asshole junkie friends were shooting some shit, you did too much and they left you for dead. If we didn't come along when we did instead of asking us what's going on, the Medical Examiner would be cutting open your chest looking for the cause of death. Have a nice day." With that rebuke, the crew of Engine 9 left the truck and took off.

I usually don't get mad at the drug-addicted patients we care for. I understand addiction. The girl in my care was a living, breathing twenty-six year old. One wrong turn and she would have been dead in the back of an old Saab. She looked as though she lived a tough life; her skin was pale and blotched, her hair damaged by too many treatments. She may have been pretty at one time, and could be again. She was slightly overweight, not from living well, probably from abusing alcohol. If she continues on this path the extra weight will slowly fade and she will become haggard. For now, she has youth on her side. She was lucky. Sometime we arrive too late, either they took too many drugs, or it was just their time and all we can do isn't enough. Sometimes the overdose victims that didn't make it reappear in my mind, their faces still and pale with the grip of death as we work on them, trying to squeeze more life out of their tired bodies. We do our best for them, breathe for them by filling their lungs with oxygen, pump their hearts for them and fill their veins with drugs to counteract the poison they've ingested. Their peaceful ride that started with a little heroin and turned drastically wrong ends in our truck, and they never know it. Sometimes they make it back, sometimes not.

I looked at the girl sitting on the stretcher in the back of my truck and marveled at the miracle of life. I was quietly thankful I don't have to add her face to the others that haunt my memories.

"How are you feeling?" I asked.

"Like an idiot. What happened to me?"

"You were with some friends. They say you overdosed on heroin."

"I'd been clean for two and a half months. I hurt my back at work and got a prescription for Vicodin. I guess that was a big mistake." She said.

"You were lucky, you could have died. Almost did actually. Don't give up on yourself; sometimes something like this can be what you need to keep you from having another relapse."

"It's so hard."

"I know."

She was back to normal for now, but the narcan has a short life and would be out of her system soon. We transported her to the ER for observation. There was a chance that she could go back into respiratory arrest. After checking her in at the triage desk, I went back to the treatment area to wash my hands. Two sinks located at the center of the room gave a great vantage point while washing. Patients filled the twenty ten-by-six foot treatment areas, separated only by curtains. Doctors and nurses converged in the middle of the room with the treatment areas circling the perimeter.

The patients have nothing to do while waiting to be treated so the center of the room becomes something like a stage, the doctors and nurses, and sometimes rescue guys providing entertainment for the bored audience.

There is not an overabundance of privacy in the ER. While drying my hands I saw another addict waving at me. I brought her here last week because she was complaining of abdominal pain. She was living in a halfway house and working for the Salvation Army. While at work she called for a rescue because of her pain. While transporting her she told me that she had been clean for six months and her life was really going well. She needed to get to the hospital because her stomach hurt so badly that she needed painkillers. I tried to talk her out of her plan, knowing that she was fooling herself into thinking a few harmless prescription painkillers wouldn't set her back. My talk didn't do much good. She told me she was here because she overdosed on heroin yesterday and got kicked out of her treatment program. Hands clean, I headed back to the truck.

THREE

We made our way back to the station to catch up on things. Usually not much happens on our days off, but if anything out of the ordinary did occur, there will be a heated discussion about it at the firehouse. The topics range from women, fires, promotions, transfers, bad meals, mistakes made, bad haircuts, sports played or watched and women; anything could come up and be fuel for discussion for days. I was told early in my career that there are three foolproof ways to communicate in this world: tele-phone, tele-graph, and tela-fireman.

The Allens Avenue fire station is located within blow-up distance of the area's fuel tank farms. Any problems resulting in an explosion will render us useless, as it is difficult to fight fire and rescue people when in the form of ashes. The station is a brick building with three floors. Mike pulled the truck onto the ramp, hit the button on the overhead door opener and backed the truck onto the apparatus floor. I saw that Engine 13 was not in the building. I hoped they were in the neighborhood shopping for lunch. Spaced between box alarms, fires, station and truck maintenance and rescue runs firefighters shop for and cook our own meals. When things get too busy there is always take-out, but we prefer to make our own.

Mike stayed on the apparatus floor to wash the truck and I headed to my office on the second floor to do the reports. I made it to the top of the stairs when the tone hit. The tone is a relatively new addition to the station having replaced the traditional fire bell. For years a loud bell would tip and everybody's heart would stop. The old bells are now coveted collectors items worth thousands of dollars. They represent an era of firefighting long gone. At one time the city had fire stations in every neighborhood. Horses hauled the steamers to the fires with the firefighters riding along or running behind. As time progressed and motorized trucks took over more ground was covered in less time. One by one the neighborhood stations were shut down and the men reassigned.

Now, the stations are equipped with state of the art PA systems. Each truck has its own tone so we know right away whose turn it is to hit the pole. The tone doesn't shock your system like the traditional bell; it was designed to gently nudge your brain into action. My brain has endured a lot of nudging over the last few years. I heard a long uninterrupted tone; Rescue 1 was being called.

1036 hrs. (10:36 a.m.)

"Engine 10 and Rescue 1 a still alarm," boomed the voice from the loudspeaker. Engine 10 is located on Broad Street, a few miles from my station. In twenty seconds, the time it should take to get to the truck from anywhere in the building, the dispatcher told us our destination.

"Engine 10 and Rescue 1, respond to 75 Lexington Avenue for a woman complaining of dizziness."

I left my reports on the desk in my office and slid the pole to the floor. My "office" is a 15'/20' space crammed with a bunk, couch, and recliner, two lockers a desk and television stand. Most of the space is covered with dust. We are overdue for a good cleaning. The rest of the upper floor consists of Engine 13's office, a luxurious space compared to the rescue room, the dorm, which the firefighters assigned to the engine share, the kitchen and what we call the day room. The kitchen is functional at best, with a series of household stoves providing the means to prepare some elaborate meals. They only last a year or two before needing replacement. Firefighters are not known for their gentle methods. Our dishwasher also takes its share of abuse and needs repair or replacement often.

The day room is the largest room on the upper floor. A widescreen television dominates one corner, two recliners and a series of couches propped in front of it. The only furniture that the city provides is two long tables, each seating six people. The chairs that went along with the tables fell into disrepair in the fifties and we are waiting for replacements. In the meantime, we bring in stuff from home or pool our money and buy things.

Every fire station in the city has a money fund which we call the "dinky." A weekly assessment of a couple of bucks is all it takes. One person manages the finances and purchases. It is a good system based on honor and is seldom abused.

Mike was rinsing the truck, only my side got washed, but half clean is better than no clean, he will finish when he has time. He shut down the hose and put it aside; we both got in and headed out the door into the bright sunlight.

Lexington Avenue is in our district, South Providence. At the turn of the century this was THE place to live. Industry was thriving, money plentiful and beautiful homes were being built. Some of the streets boast mansions on every corner. The workmanship that went into these places is phenomenal. Victorian homes dominate the streets. Ornate entryways, scrollwork and wrought iron are abundant. Stained glass fills windows. Inside, carved woodwork, spiral staircases, wood floors with inlaid patterns and ceramic tile fireplaces are among the treasures to be found. To build one of these homes today would be nearly impossible, the quality of workmanship and material no longer exists.

I am the descendant of Swedish and Irish immigrants. One great-grandfather was a carpenter; he worked on a lot of the homes in this area. He and my great-grandmother settled in Providence, worked here and raised their family. I don't know which houses he worked on, so I imagine that every one bears his stamp. I never knew him, but I feel his presence as I drive through the once grand, now poverty stricken neighborhood.

The wealthy families that filled these beautiful homes moved to areas with more privacy, their property rented and no longer given the attention it needs. I imagine that the old homes retained their dignity for a decade or two, only to fall into disrepair. As time progressed and the properties became run down, the rents decreased and the old places were no longer profitable. I've fought many fires in these houses. When their

value is less than what the insurance will cover, arson becomes an option for those with no scruples. Fires of suspicious origin happen at an alarming rate.

Many nights while smashing through a beautiful carved oak door or breaking stained glass windows with my axe to ventilate a building, I thought of the people who toiled countless hours to create such beauty. Hauling a charged 1 3/4 hose-line up a flight of mahogany stairs to hit the fire as it roared over an antique tin ceiling, the sound of the fire filling my ears, destruction all around, I was filled with helplessness and rage. Greed and instant gratification destroyed the work left by my great-grandfather, his claims of immortality reduced to ashes.

We pulled in front of the house and parked behind Engine 10. The officer, Dan walked out the front door and gave me the initial report.

"Elderly lady doesn't look so good," he told me while walking back to the engine. A lot of seasoned firefighters resent the amount of rescue runs they have to do. They would prefer to do only firefighting duty, but times have changed, and with that change came the added responsibility of Emergency Medical Services. In Providence as most cities, the fire department handles EMS. Some places have private companies working with the firefighters, not here.

Mike brought the stair chair from the back of the rescue and we walked into the house. A little Pug greeted us. He ran over to me, barked and sniffed for a while, decided I was all right then sat in a corner to observe. A young man holding a baby sat in a chair in the kitchen.

The family lived on the first floor of a three-floor house. From the look of the place, it once was a one family home, now modified to fit three or four apartments. More rent. The walls were adorned with pictures of Jesus.

"Blood pressure is 80/40 and I can't feel a pulse," said Keith, one of the firefighters from Engine 10.

"What is your name?" I asked the woman, hoping that she spoke English.

"Maria," she replied In English accentuated with Spanish tones. She added, "I've been feeling dizzy all morning and weak. I just feel terrible."

"We're going to get you to the doctor and figure out what's wrong."

I noticed that the patient was pale and covered with sweat. Her blood pressure was extremely low and her weakened state indicated a potentially serious situation. We picked her out of her bed, put her in the stair chair and transferred her to the stretcher and into the truck in about a minute.

"Is she alright?" asked the young man from the kitchen, still holding the crying infant.

"We're taking her to the hospital. How long has she been sick?" I asked.

"Just for the last fifteen minutes. She got really weak and dizzy and had to lie down. I thought she was having a heart attack or something. Which hospital are you taking her to?"

"Rhode Island."

I headed to the back of the truck where Mike had her on oxygen and hooked up to the heart monitor. Her heart rate was 174, not good. It's no wonder she felt horrible, her heart was racing out of her chest. Her blood pressure was low because her heart wasn't beating properly, merely fluttering and not providing decent pressure to fill her veins.

"Maria, are you in any pain?" I asked.

"No I just feel weak."

We started an IV and re-checked her blood pressure. I looked at the EKG and saw that her heart was still racing in a rhythm called supra ventricular tachycardia. The hospital was three minutes away. I had the choice of treating the patient with a medication called Adenosine or transporting quickly to the ER. Sometimes the adenosine is effective at slowing the heart, sometimes not. If it is effective, the heart actually stops beating for approximately thirty seconds before resuming a normal rhythm. I took into consideration the patient's age and frail condition. A team of doctors and specialists can be assembled at a minute's notice if necessary at the hospital. If I were the patient, I would rather have my heart stopped in a hospital room than the back of a truck.

"Let's go."

Mike and I stayed in back with Maria. Roland, from Engine 10 drove. The

three-minute ride went quickly. I was worried about this patient.

The triage area at RIH was in full swing. The pace was frantic; three rescues were ahead of us, their patients lying on stretchers lined up in the doorway. My patient was a priority; we passed the other people in the hall and talked to Melissa, another RN working with Ron at triage.

"I've got a seventy-four year old with a heart rate of 174, hypotensive, diaphoretic and weak. No pain at this time but complaining of dizziness." Melissa took one look at Maria and pointed to the corridor leading to the trauma rooms where the most critically ill or injured patients go. While wheeling her back I heard the hospitals P.A. system calling for a medical team to Trauma 2, one of the six trauma rooms in the ER. We headed there. While transferring Maria from our stretcher to the hospitals, the medical team began to assemble. An ER doctor, two or three trauma RN's and additional support staff were in the room before the patient. Melissa gave the report, repeating word for word what I told her at the triage desk. Maria looked worse than she did in the truck. They hooked her up to the heart monitor, checked the IV line, started another one and tried to ask her some questions. They were too late, Maria had slipped into unconsciousness, her condition critical. Her heart rhythm had gone from SVT to ventricular tachycardia, one step away from asystole and death.

In seconds, medication was given through the IV, ventilations were assisted and Maria was stabilized, breathing normally. The drugs that were administered were effective; I saw her heart return to a normal rhythm. Things happen fast in the ER.

Mike had been busy restocking and cleaning the truck. He had no idea of what just happened.

"Code 99 in the trauma room." I said.

"Who? Not Maria."

"Maria."

"Is she all right?"

"We made it here just in time. Imagine if she coded in the truck. We'd still be doing CPR."

FOUR

"I'm starving," said Mike.

"Me too, what else is new?"

We headed back to the station in hopes of having some lunch. The ride back to quarters from the hospital brings us through Providence's thriving adult entertainment section. There are other ways to get back to quarters but we chose the most colorful one. We slowed the truck as we drove by "Cheaters," a three-story pink building adorned with huge signs painted on plywood advertising "Girls, Girls, Girls." The strippers should have been coming to work right about then. We looked around but saw nothing. We passed another establishment offering a fully equipped dungeon with hourly rates. A club catering to gay men is another popular spot in the area. An adult book and novelty store completes the block. We don't get too many calls here; discretion keeps people from attracting unwanted attention. When we do get called to one of these places, it is serious; the last two times I was here the patients' died.

It was good time to call home.

"Hey babe, how are you?" I said into the cell phone, "We're driving by Cheaters right now. Naked women everywhere."

"Good for you, how is your day?"

"The usual. Are we having Easter Dinner at our house?" I asked.

"I'm not ready to give that up."

"I know, I wish I was there to help. Damn overtime"

"I'll manage."

"Have the kids help."

"Yeah, right. Can you pick up the manicotti? My mother loved the ones you got at Christmas."

"No problem, I'll pick them up as soon as I have time."

"Don't forget."

"Never happen"

"Maybe I should get them myself."

"Don't worry about a thing; they will be there on Easter morning."

"Rescue 1 and Engine 8, a still alarm," boomed the truck radio.

"I've got to go. How are you feeling?"

"Better than yesterday. Please, don't forget the manicotti."

"I won't. Love you, bye."

"Love you too."

1147 hrs. (11:47 a.m.)

"Rescue 1 and Engine 8, respond to Springfield Avenue at the elementary school for a five year old with an amputated finger."

"Rescue 1 responding," I said into the mike as I pressed the off button on the cell phone. Mike turned on the lights and siren and hit the gas. The quicker we get there, the better chance of saving the finger. Theoretically, all of our responses are emergencies, some are just more of an emergency, and we drive accordingly.

"Do you put amputated body parts directly on ice or do you wrap them first?" I asked Mike.

"I don't remember, look it up." He was focused on the road, his aloof demeanor hiding his true concern.

The elementary school was at least five minutes away so I had time to refresh my memory by reading the state protocol book. Every rescue carries one, every rescue worker should have it memorized. When you have too much time to think, you have a tendency to question your memory. I've responded to a few amputations and have always done the right thing, but it never hurts to be sure.

"The protocol says pack severed body part in sterile dressing moistened with saline, wrap in towel or plastic bag, place ice over bag," I read out loud.

"Let's hope it's not as bad as it sounds," I said to Mike as we pulled off of the highway and closed in on our destination.

"I hope it's not the middle finger, that's the most important one." he responded.

"You can always use the one on the other hand."

"But you'll never be able to pull off a double royal salute."

"Now that is a tragedy."

The radio transmitted the preliminary report from Engine 8.

"Engine 8 to fire alarm. Advise Rescue 1 we have a five-year old male with a minor laceration to his right index finger. No amputation."

"Rescue 1 received," I said into the mike as Mike slowed down.

"People should get their facts straight before they call. We could have been killed getting here," said Mike.

In the distance, the school came into view. Four giant crayons held a canopy high above the entrance. The kids that go to school here must be impressed, I certainly am. The school age population has exploded in Providence. Most of the new students don't speak English. New schools have been built to keep up with the demand.

Mike went to the rescues side compartment to get the trauma bag and I walked under the canopy into the school. I was directed to the nurse's office where firefighters, teachers and the school nurse surrounded a little boy. He looked amused by all of the attention. One of the firefighters from Engine 8 inflated a protective glove and gave it to the boy. When the bright purple gloves are inflated, the fingers resemble cow's udders. It looks pretty bizarre, which is why the kids like them so much. The boy's finger had been wrapped in sterile gauze, moistened with saline.

"He had his finger closed in a door," said Miles, one of the firefighters from Engine 8.

"Nothing seems broken, he has good movement, but there is a laceration almost completely around the finger under the first knuckle."

"There was so much blood I thought his finger was gone," added the school nurse.

"Have the parents been notified?" I asked.

"Not yet, we can't find the mother," said one of the women in the room.

"I'll need his records and we'll take him to Hasbro," I said.

Hasbro Children's Hospital is where we take all patients under sixteen. Located next to Rhode Island Hospital, it is a great facility specializing in pediatric health care.

Miles picked the boy up and carried him outside into the rescue. The school nurse accompanied us to the ER.I retrieved the necessary paperwork from the office and we were on our way.

We placed the boy, Pedro onto the stretcher. He sat on it like the king of the world being taken to his palace. I had no idea what his home life was like, but it was obvious that the attention and love that he was shown by the firefighters and school staff were enough to make him forget the pain in his finger. For a lot of these kids, the best part of their day comes when they are away from home. When responding to homes in the city I have seen living conditions unfit for animals. People unable to care for themselves bring children into the world with no idea what it takes to raise them. When child abuse or neglect is suspected we follow procedures, but have no way of finding out if our recommendations have been followed through.

Pedro looked out the back window of the rescue, his eyes wide open. From inside the truck the sirens can be heard but they are not as loud as on the outside. Things are actually peaceful during the transport.

"I can't believe how calm everybody acted," said the nurse, fidgeting on the bench seat next to Pedro. "This is my first day at this school and my first year in Providence. Nobody got very excited over this, I was the only one that did anything."

"Did you make the 911 call?" I asked.

"Nobody else would, they just stood there. If it weren't for me, they probably wouldn't even have called you. They were looking for Band-Aids."

"It probably wasn't a very good idea to tell the dispatchers that there was an amputation." I casually tried to explain to her, knowing my words are not being heard.

"Well, at least you got here fast. Everybody else was taking their time."

I sensed indignation in her words so I let it rest. She was under the impression that she alone saved the boy from severe disfigurement and possible death from blood loss. I let her bask in her moment of glory and started my report. Being lost in paperwork is a good way to avoid conversation, especially one I don't want to engage in.

At Hasbro we wheeled Pedro through the ER doors and into the waiting room. Children's books were in abundance; toys and games filled boxes next to the seats. People sat in those seats, their children either on their laps or otherwise engaged, there was plenty to keep them busy. The place was constructed with children in mind. Hand rails on the stairs come up to my knees, water fountains are at the same height. A real Fire Engine sits on the front lawn. Art by children adorns the walls of the corridors heading to the elevators. The upper floors are full of patients. I go up to those floors seldom, the suffering too much to bear. The sick kids seem to deal with leukemia, asthma, cystic fibrosis and other rare and deadly diseases better than their parents or rescue workers. They face their uncertain future with courage and dignity, seemingly baffled by the despair evident on the faces of their caregivers.

Pedro was checked in, he gave me a 'high 5' with his good hand as I left the ER.

"Enough of this, lets eat," said Mike as I opened the passenger door.

"My thoughts exactly."

We headed back to the station. The dispatchers were sending rescues all over the city for a variety of reasons. A Cranston rescue was going to Waverly Street for an intoxicated male, an East Providence rescue responded to Waterman and Ives for a car accident with no injuries, the car's occupants "just want to be checked." Rescue 3 was on the way to Smith Street for an elderly female who was dehydrated and Rescue 5 was on the scene with a two year old with a fever. Rescue 1 was going to try to get some lunch, we had a long afternoon ahead.

FIVE

Back at the station, the guys from Engine 13 had finished with lunch and were nowhere to be found. They were somewhere in the building, the engine was in the bay. Sitting on the kitchen counter were two plates wrapped in tin foil, dishes and pans were drying next to the sink.

"What do you think this is?" I asked Mike.

"I don't care, as long as it's hot, and a lot," he responded.

We opened the foil to find ravioli and sausage. The 13's must have gone to Venda, which reminded me, I had to go over there later and get the manicotti for Easter dinner at my house.

'Venda Ravioli' has been a part of the city for almost as long as the fire department. The shop is located on Federal Hill, one of my favorite parts in the city. Italian immigrants made this section their home in the early 1900's.

If you leave downtown Providence and head west onto Atwells Avenue you will enter Federal Hill. An arch stands as a gateway into the area. A giant bronze pineapple, or pinecone depending on who you talk to hangs over the street from the middle of the arch, a symbol of hospitality welcoming you in. I remember as a child spending weekends at my grandmother's house. We sometimes rode the bus to shop at The Outlet, a giant down-city department store that served as the retail center of the region before the suburban malls took over. After a few hours of shopping we would walk the mile or so from downtown to "the hill."

We walked under the arch and entered a different world. Here, people spoke Italian. The smell of garlic and onions simmering in olive oil wafting from the many restaurants' and bistros that lined the streets enhanced the mystique of the area. Shopkeepers greeted us with a smile and a tip of the cap as we walked past them on the wide sidewalk. There was no worry of crime; the streets were safe at all times. The Patriaca Family, reputed to be the head of organized crime in New England, did business in an office on the street, a small sign outside simply stating "Coin Operated Vending," a vast understatement of the influence the family had in the area.

Good manners and a bustling, friendly atmosphere surrounded us while I hauled the bags from the Outlet as my Grandmother held my free hand. If organized crime existed here, it was better than the unorganized crime of today.

We would always stop at 'Providence Cheese.'Behind the counter stood a very old man waiting to take our order. Next to him sat a tiny coffee cup with a twist of lemon floating on top of the black liquid. The meats and cheeses he had just hung in the display windows still swung from the momentum he supplied.

"One pound of grated parmesan and half a pound of ham, thinly sliced please," my grandmother would say to the man. He translated the order from English to Italian and shouted over his shoulder. The order was prepared by hand, meat sliced with sharp knives, cheese grated the old fashioned way, with hand held graters, by a group of Italian speaking ladies "in the back." The order was filled, money exchanged, the next person in line waited on.

Venda Ravioli was next, two doors down.

"Two dozen cheese," my grandmother said which put the ladies in the back into action. The pasta would be rolled flat, filled with cheese and cut into squares. The ladies never stopped talking and laughing as they want about their work. The ravioli was placed on wax paper, put into a cardboard box then wrapped with a red ribbon. We paid then headed home to make the sauce (the Italians call it gravy!) and had a feast.

"This ravioli tastes like homemade." said Mike, a dribble of "gravy" rolling down his chin.

"It is." I answered, reluctantly returning to the present.

"Rescue 1 and Engine 10, a still alarm." The voice in the loudspeaker helped bring me back.

1339 hrs (1:39 p.m.)

Rescue 1 and Engine 10, respond to 9 Peace Street at St. Josephs Hospital for a maternity."

We re-wrapped our unfinished lunch with the tinfoil and put it aside for later. We had staved off the hunger for a while, but weren't really satisfied. We were back in the rescue with lights flashing and sirens blaring a minute later. What little lunch we had was going to have to get us through the afternoon.

"Did you call a rescue for Amy when she was ready to deliver?" I asked Mike.

"What are you crazy?" he responded, "I put her in the car and drove her to the hospital. We had nine months to get ready, it wasn't an emergency until we got to the delivery room."

"How much blood did she lose?"

"Almost two liters. I couldn't even see her for three hours after the delivery, she was in intensive care."

"How are they doing now?"

"Perfectly healthy," he responded like the proud papa, "we wanted to have six kids, two might have to do it."

"Two is enough. Your whole life will revolve around them from now on. I wonder if bringing up boys will be any easier than girls, my two are still driving me crazy."

"Speaking of girls, how are the wedding plans going?" asked Mike.

"Right on schedule, I guess. Cheryl is doing all of the work; I haven't had time to do anything. Danielle as usual has every detail planned. It's funny, all I do is walk her down the aisle, but I get all the credit."

"That's the way it should be."

We pulled in front of St. Joseph's hospital as Engine 10 walked out with two women, a mother and daughter, the younger of the two looking ready to deliver a child right there.

"Contractions twelve minutes apart, water not broken, a real emergency," said Dan.   He helped the girl and her mother into the rescue. The fire department sends an engine company with the rescue when called for a maternity response. We have delivered thousands of babies over the years. Years ago, if somebody called 911 for assistance for a pregnant woman, delivery was imminent. Now, we are called for rides to the hospital for check-ups.

Mike placed the girl on the stretcher, her mother on the bench seat next to her. It didn't give us a lot of room to work. I sat in the Captains chair at the head of the patient. Mike started to get her vital signs and I began the interview.

"What is your name"?

"No comprehende' English." She said with a smile. I look to her mother for help but she smiled also and shook her head no.

"ID." I held my thumb and forefinger as if holding a card. The girl smiled and reached into her purse to retrieve a medical card with her name and date of birth on it. The State has a program that provides medical coverage to the poor. I see these cards a lot during the course of a day.

I copied the information while Mike tried to communicate with them.

"Blood pressure 148/90, pulse 98, pulsox 98%. Contractions about ten minutes apart. She was at her doctor's office when the contractions began, he called us for a ride to Woman and Infants. This is her first pregnancy, no complications, due date ten days."

"How did you find all that out?" I asked, his knowledge of Spanish is only slightly better than mine.

"It's my job, man." He headed to the front of the truck to drive leaving me mystified in the back with two Spanish-speaking women. They were all smiles, their happiness contagious as I smile with them. An old Springsteen' song accompanied us to Woman and Infants; I filled out the rest of the report on the way, humming along with 'MyHometown.'

SIX

"Let's finish lunch," I said to Mike as we left Woman and Infants.

"That sausage is giving me gas," he replied, the evidence pungently filled the cab of the rescue.

I looked over at him, saw that he was pleased by his latest contribution to global warming and said, "What's the matter with you, you couldn't have left that outside?"

"I wanted to share it with you," he replied.

"Five hundred people on the job and I get you."

"I've got more bad news," he said while maneuvering the busy lunchtime traffic surrounding the hospitals."I'm bidding Engine 15."

The day I dreaded finally arrived. My heart sank to the floor of the rescue, my emotional response to this news stronger than I ever had imagined. I've had other partners since being promoted, but Mike and I were like brothers. His presence made an always difficult and sometimes impossible job bearable. Things had been going so well I hadn't thought about losing another partner; vital to your well being and sanity on a rescue truck in Providence. I was happy for him; Engine 15 is a busy truck that sees a lot of fire. I've told everybody I work rescue with the same thing, make sure you do time on a fire truck before it is too late. When our days are closing in and we look back at our lives, what we will be most proud of will probably be the years spent as a firefighter. I want everybody to experience the thrill I've felt while battling a fully involved house fire. There is nothing like strapping on a Scott, grabbing a line and facing what most men fear. Working to the brink of exhaustion, then finding a little more when needed and ultimately beating the beast is priceless.

"Rescue 5 a still alarm."

"I hope that's not in our district." I say, hoping to make it back to the station, choosing to ignore Mike's news until I've had time to sort things out.

"Rescue 5 respond to 1035 Broad Street at the pay phone for an intoxicated male."

Our district. Damn.

1355 hrs (1:55 p.m.)

"Darryl." We said simultaneously. I keyed the mike.

"Rescue 1 to Fire Alarm, we're coming in service from Women and Infants, we'll handle."

"Message received, Rescue 1, you have it. Rescue 5 disregard."

Darryl calls 911 every day, sometimes twice a day. He's done it for years. One of the numerous homeless alcoholics living in the city, he abuses the health care system. His survival mechanism incorporates the cities rescues, emergency rooms, homeless shelters and the state penitentiary system.

As we approached 1035 Broad Street I saw a human form crumpled on the sidewalk, lying under a pay phone. A convenience store sat fifty feet from the street; the stores customers had to step around him to get inside. We stopped the truck and gloved up.

"Darryl! Wake up, it's time to go." I said, nudging him with my foot. The store's patrons barely glanced at us, they have seen this show hundreds of times.

"Come on, let's go," added Mike. "There's a seafood buffet waiting at the hospital in your honor, everybody is waiting for you. Drinks, entertainment, you name it. Today is Darryl day in Providence, the Mayor is going to give you the keys to the City."

"Gimmee a sandwich," is all we got out of Darryl.

Some days he can walk, others he has to be carried. We got on both sides of him, helped him to his feet and assisted him to the door of the truck. We let him sit on the bench seat; he hadn't lost his bowels or bladder yet.

"Aren't you tired of this?" I asked him on the way to the ER.

"Fuck you."

That went well. We rode to the hospital together in the back of the rescue, physically close yet worlds apart.

The smell of Darryl mixed with Mike's contribution from earlier filled the truck. I wondered if I was breathing contaminated molecules. I turned on the ventilation system in back, the sound of the fan a comforting hum.

We have a picture on the door of my office of Saddam Hussein, disheveled and filthy with a long straggly beard, after his capture. Darryl could be his double. Prison tattoos adorn his forearms, the blue ink faded but legible. One says "Mom" the other arm "Love."

"What's with the new clothes, did you hit the lottery?" I asked him. His taste runs toward dirty sweatshirts and jeans, today he had on a nice pair of khaki pants and a button down shirt. He even wore shoes and socks rather than his usual sneakers. Darryl mumbled some unintelligible grunts and passed out while sitting on the seat. I used to wonder how he could be conscious one minute, then comatose the next. Recently I found out his secret;

he opens a newspaper vending machine with fifty cents that he panhandled from somebody and steals the entire stack. He takes his papers a few blocks away and sells them to people heading into a convenience store. When he has made enough for some cheap vodka, he ditches what papers are left in the trash and buys a bottle. Some days a half pint will do, others a quart. The next step is to go to his favorite phone booth, call 911 and claim there is an intoxicated person at the pay phone. The dispatchers know what is going on, but have to send us. If they refuse, he will continue to call, claim he is having chest pains or has been assaulted. He then guzzles the bottle of vodka. He drinks it strait from the bottle in about thirty seconds. If we are in a different part of the city when the call comes in and have a delayed response, the vodka has time to work its magic and he is unconscious when we arrive on the scene. If we get there quickly, he is still coherent for a little while, then lapses into a drunken stupor. Eventually, he will kill himself. Some days when we get to him he is so far gone that we have to start an IV and intubate. His liver is shot, his heart ready to give up and his brain damaged to the brink of retardation. The health care providers have given up hope of rehabilitation, every chance was given to him, yet he refuses to follow through with his treatment. I wish I could say that I feel sorrow or pity toward him but I truly don't. When he dies another homeless alcoholic will take his place, just like he took the place of the last one that died. The real tragedy is that he and those like him are allowed to squander the limited resources of the health care system. He is on full disability, and receives a check each month from the taxpayers to spend any way he chooses. He chooses to drown himself in vodka while we pick up the tab. If I sound bitter, that is because I am.

"Mike, you're going to have to get a stretcher." I said as we backed into the rescue bay at RIH. "Our patient is no longer with us."

"He died?"

"Kind of."

I waited for the stretcher. A few moments later, Mike wheeled a hospital stretcher to the side door of the rescue and we hauled Darryl onto it.

"Why don you guys leave him in the woods?" Domingo asked as we wheel him past.

"He be better off livin wit the animals." He continued.

Ron saw the patient and rushed over.

"Get him in the back, we need him right away!" he said, a look of relief on his face.

"What's going on around here?" Mike asked.

"I'll tell you in a minute." Ron wheeled Darryl into one of the back rooms of the ER.

My skin felt disgusting, I wanted to take a shower but a good hand scrubbing had to do. The sinks in the middle of the treatment area served as my shower.

The ER was in full swing, a four-hour wait for patients seeking routine emergency care. Critical patients are seen immediately. I took a look around the room as I scrubbed. I never fail to be impressed with this place; the volume of patients would overwhelm most health care facilities. RIH is the only Level 1 trauma center in the area. Patients are cared for, tests ordered; illness diagnosed and medicated, bones set, lacerations stitched and everybody cared for at levels of professionalism from the doctors and nursing staff that you can't find anywhere else. Controlled chaos fills the halls between the patients, the frantic pace exhausting to watch. Trauma and medical teams are routinely called to trauma alley. The trauma teams don't sit around waiting for trauma or life threatened patients, they provide quality care to the hundreds of routine patients that seek it here. When the speaker blares out "Trauma team to Trauma 1," they drop what they are doing and go. They have no idea what to expect, a gunshot wound, amputation, electrocution, anything could be waiting for them. They finish the job in trauma alley, sometimes with heartbreaking results then pick up where they left off.

"He came back just in time," said Ron as I returned to the triage desk.

"What was the rush?" I asked. "I've never seen Darryl go to the back so fast."

"That guy look familiar?" Ron asked me. He indicated with a nod of the head a man leaving the ER through the waiting room door.

"Kind of."

"Rescue brought him here last night around the same time as Darryl. They found him intoxicated at the Foxy Lady. We put them in the same detox room. Darryl was released first and took his roommates clothes.

"Ever the opportunist," I said.

"Maybe that guy is still wearing Darryl's undies," said Mike as we walked out of the ER.

Mike and I headed back to the truck and into the city. We drove past the man possibly wearing Darryl's underwear as he made his way back to whatever life he led.

I'm going to miss Mike.

SEVEN

"Mike, do you want to work tonight?" It was the division chief calling on the department cell phone. Every inch of me screams no, but I say "Yes sir."

"How about Leclaire?" the chief asked

"Mike, do you want a callback tonight?" I asked him.

"Only if I see monkeys fly out of my ass."

"He says no, sir."

I'll be going to Rescue 3 in the city's north end. Captain Fortes hurt his back a while ago and the department has been filling his spot with overtime. Good for me.

"You shouldn't work so much overtime," said Mike.

"You should work more overtime," I replied.

"But look at how well rounded I am," he continued. "You're a burned out shell. You need to spend more time with your family."

"I know." I keyed the mike and went back in service.

1458 hrs. (2:58 p.m.)

"Rescue 1, head over to 20 Grand Street for a woman with difficulty walking."

Twenty Grand Street is another high rise apartment building inhabited by elderly and disabled people. The people who live there have established their own community where English is seldom spoken. Occasionally somebody's children or grandchildren will be visiting and we can use them as a translator, for the most part we are on our own. The language barrier is something that we deal with daily. I communicate with sign language and a few Spanish words, my patients respond likewise. Experience has taught me how to treat patients with very little verbal communication, a heart attack looks the same every language, you just have to recognize the signs and symptoms.

A security guard buzzed us into the lobby and we headed toward the elevator. It was small, we made the stretcher fit by folding up the back. I hate being crowded into these elevators, the things I have seen crawling on their walls make my skin crawl. A resident tried to get in with us, I told him to wait for the next one and the door closed on him. He was pissed, I think he swore at us in Spanish.

"What's the matter with that guy?" Mike asked.

"He likes your ass and wanted to get a little closer," I responded.

"Well, why didn't you let him in?" he said, "I could have used a little stimulation."

"Maybe he'll be waiting for us on the way down," I said as the elevator door opened and we made our way down the corridor. Dead bugs trapped in the fluorescent light fixtures cast shadows on the doors that lined the hallway, some of which were decorated, most were bare. What lies behind those doors is a mystery. Pungent aroma's seeped out giving some clues; somebody was baking, someone else hadn't bathed in years. You never know what to expect until the door opens. Our patient was behind the last door.

"What's the matter?" I asked the lady sitting on a couch in her parlor. Her place was well kept and nicely furnished. Her kitchen was to our left as we entered, candies sat in a bowl on the table.

"I've been throwing up since yesterday," she said in English with a faint southern drawl. "I'm so weak I can't make it to the bathroom."

"Let's get you to the hospital then, you look awful." I told her. Her name was Ethyl. She was dressed in red pajamas, top and a bottom with yellow fuzzy slippers on her feet and a bright yellow scrungy holding her hair in a bun. As sick as she was, she brightened the room. We helped her to the stretcher, locked up her place and made our way to the truck. Ethel rode in the stretcher and greeted everybody we passed in the hallway and lobby in Spanish by their first names. They all looked concerned and wished her well.

"You are the only person that I've met here that speaks English," I told her as we loaded the stretcher with her on it into the back of the rescue. "You could be the Ambassador!"

"Not so many speak English," she explained. "When I moved here from Columbia, South Carolina fifty years ago there weren't many Hispanic people at all. Me and the rest of the black folks are a minority around here now. Times have changed but people are still the same."

"Do you speak Spanish?" I asked.

"Just enough to get by," she responded. I wonder how much that was.

"I would have taken myself to the hospital but I don't drive. My granddaughter was going to take me but she said I should call 911 and she would meet me there."

"Why don't you drive?" I asked.

"Never did, I can't even ride a bike. The Good Lord provided me with legs and that is what I use."

Ethyl's vital signs were stable; we transported to RI Hospital without any medical procedures. She was probably dehydrated from throwing up and just needed fluids. We got to the hospital at around 3:00. The traffic was brutal; shift change brings chaos to the area around the hospital. Finally we pulled into the rescue bay and got Ethel checked in. This was a routine call for us; we welcome the break from the serious runs and drunks that we usually encounter. Ethel was a beautiful person; it is good to know that such people still exist in the city. I went back to the truck to call Cheryl and tell her about Ethyl.

EIGHT

"Hello."

"Hey babe, what are you doing?" I ask.

"I just finished cleaning the house, I'm headed out to the store, how are you?"

"Great. I'm working at Rescue 3 tonight."

"I wish you didn't have to work so much overtime. I feel responsible. If I was still working you could go back to Engine 9 and we could have a normal life."

"I wish you didn't have Multiple Sclerosis but you do and nothing is going to change that. I know that you do what you can so don't worry about it. Thank God I love this stupid job, if I didn't I would really be miserable instead of just acting like I am. I just had a great old lady in the truck. She was sick as a dog but managed to tell me all about her life in South Carolina. She moved up here fifty years ago with her family and has made a pretty good life for herself."

"Why is she going to the hospital?"

"She's sick."

"I know she's sick you idiot, what's the matter with her?"

"Nothing a little IV fluid won't cure." I said.

"Call me later."

"Will do. Love you, bye."

"Love you too."

We made it back to the station at 3:30. Mike stayed on the apparatus floor to finish washing the truck; I headed upstairs to finish my reports. Every rescue run is carefully documented. We fill out a State EMS form in triplicate before we leave the hospital. Information concerning the patient's medical history, allergies to medicine and medicines taken are provided on the form. We give a detailed narrative pertaining to the patient's present condition, record vital signs and treatment we have provided before the triage nurse signs the form. The hospital gets a copy; I take the rest back to the station with me.

At my desk, I transposed the information onto the hard drive of my computer and filed the hard copies. The EMS Chief picks the reports up weekly. Any rescue report needed can be found in minutes. A lot of lawyers request the forms for cases they are preparing. Occasionally we get dragged into court to testify. I've yet to have to appear, but I have heard some horror stories about what happens. The wheels of justice turn slowly, we can be called to testify on cases years after the incident and be expected to remember the smallest details.

The guys were gathered around the sitting room torturing each other. My appearance gives them a new target.

"I didn't know there was a full solar eclipse happening today," says Captain Healy, the man in charge of Engine 13.

"There's not, Mike's head just passed the window," says Steve as he looks up from the paper he is reading.

"Doesn't your neck get tired holding up all that weight?" asks Jay.

"His head may be big but there is nothing but air inside." The Captain contributes.

My head really isn't that big. The helmet I was issued years ago in the academy was too small and I have never heard the end of it.

"The Chief called," I said to Captain Healy, "they've perfected the super stretch spandex material for your pants, they should be ready any time."

"They're waiting for a new machine that fastens giant waistbands to tiny legs," said Steve.

"I thought they ran out of material after making his last pair," added Jay.

"Rescue 1 a still alarm."

"Five bucks for lunch," said Steve as the loudspeaker continued to blare.

"Rescue 1 respond to 14 Lennox Avenue for a child with a laceration to his head."

I put the five on the table and headed back out, leaving the guys to their own devices.

1646 hrs. (4:46 p.m.)

This was Mike's last run for the day; I had twenty-five hours to go. We were heading into a rough section of the city. Providence may be the Renaissance City to some, just don't tell that to the people that live in this neighborhood. The Renaissance passed without a backward glance.

A gang of young guys stood around the front of the house, dressed in jerseys, gold jewelry, jeans and expensive sneakers. The jerseys they wore are a status symbol in the neighborhood and cost up to three hundred dollars each.

I remembered one of these guys from an ugly incident on this street last summer. A street brawl had erupted; ultimately one of the fighters was stabbed. The crowd that gathered was emotionally charged as they watched their friend die before their eyes. Some franticly dialed 911 from their cell phones expecting us to rush to their aid. They waited for what must have seemed to them an abnormally long time, but in actuality were only minutes. The fire department has procedures in place which direct us to wait for the police to secure a violent incident before we move in. This night there were no police on the scene and a large crowd had formed. Firefighters have been attacked by hostile crowds. Engine 10 had been dispatched along with us and slowly approached the scene from one side, we approached from the other. The victim's friends didn't think we moved fast enough. It is our nature to help people, we just don't want to get killed along the way. Cautiously we moved in. As I was getting the stretcher out of the back of the rig, one of the guys now standing in front of the house accosted me.

"If he dies, you die."

"You stupid bastard," I told him, focused on the patient and annoyed by the interruption, "your friend is bleeding to death and you have to bust my balls. Get out of the way or your friend will die on those steps." He relented, realizing we were the best chance he had. The rest of the crowd shouted racial epithets and stood in our way, six middle aged white guys stood out in this neighborhood where we normally don't belong. The tension in the air was thick. I continued to make progress toward the patient. The guys from Engine 10 kept the hostile crowd under control somehow and helped load the patient, a twenty year old male with a two inch stab wound to his abdomen and his shoulder sliced wide open onto the stretcher and into the truck. Once we gained control of the scene the crowd let us work. In two minutes we had the patient stabilized and on the way to the ER. The police showed up as we sped away.

The victim was critical, his wounds life threatening. We got him to the ER where the doctors saved his life, and possibly mine.

Mike pulled the truck in front of the house, the gang gave us some space as we walked past them up a flight of stairs and into a second floor apartment. They were not friendly but we have earned their respect.

The apartment was filthy. The victim, an adorable three-year old boy wearing only a diaper sat on an old chair, the stuffing falling to the floor from rips in the upholstery. He had a small bump on his head, no other sign of injury.

"He was running around and ran right into a wall," said a twenty year old guy dressed in a sleeveless t-shirt and jeans. "I told his mother not to call you, he'd be fine."

"I'm going to check him out." I said. "What is his name?"

"We call him 'Gordo,'" said the man, grinning. Many more people were in the apartment, watching us with wary eyes.

I got down to the boy's level and said, "Gordo, are hurt anywhere?" He looked me in the eye and shook his head no.

Though the living conditions were deplorable, it seemed that these people loved the boy and looked out for his interests to the best of their ability. Gordo seemed comfortable and unafraid. This is the lifestyle these people are used to, they are comfortable with it. Because I disagree with it doesn't make me right. Gordo was fine, no need for transport. Some people grow up in houses like these and become successful. Most stay and bring more kids into a world that they cannot escape.

There was no need for us to transport "Gordo."

The day shift was done. We headed back to the station, Mike going home, myself headed to the North End of the city and Rescue 3. I can't believe I'm losing Mike to Engine 15. I want to ask him to stay but don't want to put any pressure on him. His decision to leave the truck put me in a tough spot.

Before Mike was assigned with me I seriously had considered leaving the rescue division and going back to my old assignment; firefighter on Engine 9. It would mean a reduction in rank and cut in pay as well as lost overtime. Mike was like the cavalry coming over the hill, just in the nick of time. The relentless calls for help never end. I was tired of helping people, most of who refuse to help themselves. During my days off I found it harder and harder to sleep and snapped at my family. The people I worked with were good at what they did, but I never felt a bond with them. They were just people to work with, I never was able to share with them my downward spiral. Mike changed all that. He helped me see the job from a new perspective and made it fun again. I could talk to him as a friend. I didn't want to work with anybody else.

When I thought back of the day's events I felt a sense of accomplishment. I was a little tired, but couldn't worry about that, I had a long night ahead.

The ride to the other end of the city takes about twenty minutes, depending on rush hour traffic. Some days when traffic is light I can make the trip in ten. I enjoyed the ride, listened to talk radio and relaxed for the first time all day. It was only twenty minutes, but to be away from the rescue and all that comes with it was a welcome relief. I needed a little time to clear my head.

PART II

PART II

NINE

I steered my wagon off of the highway and turned into the driveway of the Branch Avenue Fire Station. I started my career here, running with Engine 2 and Ladder 7. The station itself is similar to the Allens Avenue barn, only twice as large. I saw a lot of fire while stationed there and learned some important things about station life and fighting fires. Just as important, I made some life long friends that I look forward to seeing whenever I work overtime on Rescue 3. It is a homecoming of sorts whenever I enter this building.

I pulled my car around the side of the building and drove into an underground parking garage. This station also has three levels, the basement parking garage, the apparatus floor in the middle and the living quarters on top. The indoor parking is a nice perk that most stations don't have. Guys stationed here have the cleanest cars in the city. As I walked up the stairs I saw that Rescue 3's bay was empty, giving me some more time away from the stress of being on call. I said quick hello's to some of the guys as I passed them on my way up the stairs. Change of shift is a busy time at the station. Twelve people coming, twelve going.

Rescue 3's office is twice as large as Rescue1's, but that doesn't make it better. Even though I spent years here I feel like a stranger in this room. A desk and bunk fill one side of the room, a bureau with a TV on top stands at the end of the bunk. Years ago one of the officers brought in a sectional sofa from home and put it in Rescue 3's office. He has retired, but the couch is still there. It beckons; I'm asleep in seconds.

1745 hrs. (5:45 p.m.)

"Rescue 3 a still alarm"
It seemed that I had just shut my eyes.

"Rescue 3; respond to 57 Pleasant Street for a man bleeding on the sidewalk, stage for police"

I got up from the couch and slid the pole to the apparatus floor. The rescue would be driving past the station on the way to this run. The guys working the day shift must be ready to go home, I'd catch them on the ramp. A new guy, Renato waited outside, my partner for the night. I didn't know him that well and heard that he had very little rescue experience, but a great attitude. I'll take a great attitude over an experienced bad one any day. Renato introduced himself and shook my hand and the night was under way.

I saw Rescue 3 heading toward us from North Main Street. When they saw us they turned off the lights and sirens to not draw attention. We did the change of shift on the ramp with the engine still running. I was in a new truck with a new partner, ready for whatever the night had to offer.

Pleasant Street is anything but. Three streets away from the station and you would think you had entered another world. There are rumors of extensive drug dealing going on in this area. The tenement houses are in disrepair, broken windows, peeling paint and years of neglect stifle what beauty may have once thrived here. It appears that those who now live here have abandoned all hope.

Graffiti adorned the pavement, fences and houses, broken glass, and spent bullet casings littered the ground. Lawlessness pervades the area, passed from one generation to the next.

We drove from North Main into the thick of things. A young man leaned against a curb, bleeding. A crowd of neighborhood kids surrounded him. From my vantage point, the scene looked relatively safe, kids on bicycles circled the area and nobody appeared openly hostile. There was a pretty young nurse helping the bleeding boy, I was worried for her safety.

"Head up there, Renato." He gunned the motor and closed in. I keyed the mike, "Rescue 3 on scene, no police."

"What happened here?" I asked as we got out of the truck and walked over to the victim.

"A bunch of niggers kicked his ass and stole his jewelry," responded a young girl of fifteen or so. She was Hispanic. Racism is alive and well in Providence. They don't need white people to keep the tradition alive.

"I was driving home from work and noticed a gang of kids beating him up," the nurse explained. "He didn't lose consciousness but he has a pretty good laceration to the back of his head."

"Thanks for helping," I said. "This is a pretty rough section; you could have gotten yourself killed."

"They're just kids," she responded. She was right, they were just kids. I wondered if she realized that some of these kids carried loaded weapons.

At one time African Americans dominated this street. In recent years the Hispanic population has exploded. At times I don't see much love between the two groups.

"Do you know what day it is?" I asked the victim. He didn't. Some days I don't know the answer to that question either so I asked another.

"Do you know who the president is?"

"Bill Clinton." He responded.

Close. I was asking simple questions to determine the severity of his head injury. If the person is oriented to his surroundings, his level of consciousness can be determined.

"Do you know who you are?"

He looked at me with bewildered eyes.

"Renato, get the board and grab a collar. I think he has a concussion."

Renato got the necessary supplies from the truck and I got the stretcher from the back. We had the patient lie flat on his back after applying the cervical collar. With help from the nurse on scene and some of the kids in the crowd, we loaded him onto the stretcher and into the truck. A crowd had gathered and watched us work. They were not openly hostile, but I sensed tension rising. There is always the risk of violence erupting, especially at violent incidents. The boy's girlfriend came along in the back, quietly observing as we did our job. I thanked the nurse and watched as she returned to her car then closed the rescue doors and got to work. I put an oxygen mask over the patients face and adjusted the flow to ten liters. Renato placed three EKG leads in the appropriate places and ran a strip. I placed a blood pressure cuff on the patient's right arm while Renato looked for a vein to establish an IV on his left. A pulsoximeter lead was put over a finger of his right hand and a reading recorded before the cuff inflated. Renato probably needed the practice so I let him attempt the IV. Young people in good shape are easy to stick and good confidence builders. He got it on the first try. The IV line was attached to the end of the catheter, the flow set, the line secured and we were ready to go. I wrote the report:

Pt. Found semi-conscious leaning against wall, contusion and small laceration to back of head. Pt. Punched and kicked by numerous assailants, no loc. IV est, 18 G. L. a/c. B/P 188/110, spo2 98%. Sinus tach at 124. 10 L. 02 adm. via mask, board and collar applied, transported to Hasbro.

I heard some commotion on the outside and took a look out of the rear window. A middle-aged woman was at the door of the rescue yelling in Spanish. Renato opened the back door. They talked for a while until she settled down. Renato translated for me.

"I told her what happened. She's going to follow us to Hasbro."

"Tell her to meet us there; it's dangerous following a rescue."

Renato translates.

"She said she'll meet us there."

I would have bet my house that she would be right behind us as we transported.

Two police officers approached the scene as we left.I gave them a brief summary of the assault before taking off.The kid in the rescue was in a tough spot. If he decided to press charges retribution could be swift and heavy. If he takes matters into his own hands he runs the risk of getting involved in a cycle of violence that only ends badly. If he does nothing, he will be considered easy prey. He has some hard choices to make with no easy answer. Getting out of the neighborhood could be his only alternative. I am thankful I don't have to put my kids in the position to make those decisions. Just getting through adolescence is hard enough. He has big problems that need to be solved.

Traffic was light, rush hour was over. I looked out of the rear windows of the rescue and saw a car ten feet behind us with the emergency flashers activated.

"Are you alright?" I asked the girl.

"Just upset. I just moved to that neighborhood yesterday. I can't believe this happened. My boyfriend was just visiting. He didn't need this."

"Where did you move from?" I asked.

"Potters Ave."

Potters Avenue is in South Providence, Pleasant Street the North End. There is a little gang war going on between the two neighborhoods. The kids getting shot don't tell me much, but we have an idea of what is going on.

"Isn't there some bad blood between those two neighborhoods?" I asked.

"There is but I don't get involved in that stuff. Neither does he." She pointed to the boy on the stretcher. He was doing fine, vitals stable, heart rate a little high but nothing life threatening.

I had a feeling that these two kids would make it out of their present situation. The streets that they live on are the roughest around. If they don't get involved with the gangs and all that comes with it they will have a chance. If they are seduced by the "hood life" they will spend the rest of their lives in places like this. There isn't a lot of hope for the future on these streets; the present is pretty bleak also.

Renato backed the rescue into the bay at Hasbro, the boy's mother right behind us. The waiting room was packed. Every seat was full and little kids littered the floor. People waited six hours to be seen. My patient went directly to the back and into a trauma room. There the trauma team assembled and started his care. The boy's girlfriend waited outside of the doors next to the boy's mother. They did a great job of pretending the other didn't exist.

TEN

"If those kids can get out of here and go away to college, I think they will be alright." I said to Renato.

We traversed the city from the south side back to the north end. This was my favorite time of night. The workforce had made their way home, the people who live here were busy with dinner and things were quiet. The thoroughfare toward the station has made a remarkable transformation in the last decade. The truck hugged the Providence River for the first part of the ride. Eventually, the Providence converges with the Moshassock and Woonasquatucket rivers. Water Place Park is the newest addition to the city's numerous parks and museums. Providence was once listed in the Guinness book of World Records for having the widest bridge in the world. The beautiful waterway was covered by concrete, rebar and gravel giving the illusion of land. Underneath the bridge flowed what now is heralded as one of the most beautiful parts of the city. The ugly roadway has been torn down. Venetian style bridges now cross the rivers; a gondolier can often be seen plying the waterways. What once was a polluted mass of dead water moving under a dying city is now a less polluted waterway boasting restaurants, park benches and festivals such as an event called "Waterfire."

Twelve times a year, bonfires are lit in the middle of the three rivers on cauldrons created just for that purpose. One hundred bonfires burn in the center of the moving water, opera music is piped into the park and thousands of people come downtown to share the serenity. Artists, performers and giant puppets known as the Big Nazu mingle with folks out for a leisurely stroll. People put aside their fears and differences and come together to embrace the serenity and bask in the mutual admiration of the best the city has to offer. Even if only for a short while, it is time well spent.

Rhode Island School of Design has built dorms and classrooms along the route. Students from RISD and other local colleges make up a large part of the city's population. Every year, as summer grudgingly gives way to fall, new students converge on the city with their families, eager and alive with anticipation. The city invites them, welcoming them with open arms showing the best the city has to offer, conveniently bypassing the ugly underbelly of Providence. Some kids look for housing away from the dorms and end up living in triple-deckers surrounded by drug addicts, prostitutes and murderers. Proud parents, heads filled with propaganda supplied by the savvy marketing people employed by the city and colleges leave their kids and head to their homes in Jersey, New York and elsewhere, hope mixed with trepidation, yet secure in the knowledge that they have done their best to prepare their children for adulthood. The kids are eager to experience their freedom and explore their new surroundings, fearless and full of bravado. Their lives having just begun they experience for the first time the joy of discovery. Too many make it into the back of my rescue, beaten senseless and robbed not only of material possessions, but their innocence as well.

Some take it in stride, others fail and head back home, not ready for the college experience. The ones that stay blend in with the schools personality. They show up in the fall looking like average kids. By spring they have been transformed into eccentric RISD students, pink hair, black clothes, tattoos, piercings and a host of other improvements that their parents must love.

Days on Rescue go by quickly. I showed up for work twelve hours ago, it seemed like half that. We made it back to the station at 6:30. Renato showed me his new car. I missed it when I parked in the downstairs garage. A 2004 Lexus sat in the corner, glistening under the fluorescent lights. My old Toyota wagon was parked on the other side of the garage looking dull and tired under the same lights. The drivers of these vehicles looked a little like their cars; me, old and tired, Renato, new and fresh. Oh well. Renato stayed in the garage to wax the Lexus, I went upstairs to check on my family.

"Hey Babe, what are you doing?" I was sitting at the desk in Rescue 3's office, talking on my cell phone.

"Making topiaries for the wedding, how was your day?"

"Not bad. I'm at Branch Ave. Renato speaks Spanish."

"Who's Renato?"

"A guy from the last school. He's brand new but seems pretty cool."

"That should help."

"I guess, but the bad news is, Mike is leaving rescue. I was hoping he'd stay."

"What are you going to do?"

"I don't know. I love the job, but without Mike I don't want to do it anymore. He made it bearable. You know, he never complained about anything, kept me sane when I thought I couldn't take it anymore."

"Why don't you tell him?" Cheryl thinks like a woman. God forbid men let other men know how they really feel.

"I can't do that. It wouldn't be fair to him. You know what really sucks? I'm actually pretty good at this. I loved fighting fires but I never got the same satisfaction from that as I do on the rescue truck. I actually do some good every day."

"You were a pretty good firefighter from what I hear," she says.

"I guess, but there are four hundred good firefighters on the job. Not that many are good at rescue. I want to stay, but without the right partner it's unbearable. The amount of calls make it almost impossible to keep a good attitude."

"Why don't they get rid of some of the fire trucks and add rescues?"

"We have a good fire force. You can't rob Peter to pay Paul. I don't know what I'm going to do. I just can't see myself riding rescue with somebody who hates it."

"I'm sure you'll think of something. Did you get to Venda?"

Shit. "No, I'll get there tomorrow."

"You forgot."

"No I didn't, I figured tomorrow would be more convenient."

"Bullshit."

"Right."

"Rescue 3 a still alarm." Just in the nick of time.

"I've got a run, I'll call you later."

"Be careful."

'Love you, bye."

1946 hrs. (7:46 p.m.)

Rescue 3 and Engine 12, Respond to Hawkins and Admiral for a reported shooting."

I key the mike. "Rescue 3 on the way."

Renato was in the truck, engine running and emergency lights flashing. The overhead door opened and we headed into the night. Cars pulled to either side of us as we made our way to our destination. We had about four minutes before arriving on scene.

"I've never been to a shooting," said Renato.

"Be careful. Try to get the victim to the hospital as quickly as possible. IV, O2 and an EKG are mandatory. Use a lot of towels to control the bleeding and get away from the scene as quickly as possible. Keep your eyes open, sometimes the crowd turns on us."

The adrenaline rush en-route to a shooting is similar to that of responding to a fire. Not only is there a victim at the destination, your own life could be in jeopardy as well. We flew out of the station toward the incident, monitoring the police radio all the way. After a few minutes Engine 12 gave the initial report.

"Engine 12 to Fire Alarm!" I could tell from the voice on the radio that this was the real thing. Not panicked by any means, but urgency usually not heard from a seasoned fire officer.

"Confirmed shooting, police on scene, two victims, send another rescue, expedite."

We stepped it up and made it on scene in three minutes. The door to an apartment building stood wide-open letting in the cold air. Police were everywhere, their radio's blaring indecipherable messages. A firefighter from Engine 12 directed us through the front door of the apartment building down a long hallway and into a crowded room. A crowd had congregated inside, police and partygoers. A smoky haze enveloped the area giving it a dreamlike aura. I saw a young black man slouched in an old wingback chair, barely breathing, frothy sputum escaping from his nose and mouth. His girlfriend, hysterical, stood behind the dying man screaming. I stood in front of the two; assessing the victim's condition before asking the firefighter if anybody was in worse condition. He indicated a man in the rear bedroom was shot also. I walked away from the two in the chair toward to the rear of the apartment. The girl who was screaming moments ago directed her anger at me suddenly jumped from behind the chair and attacked me. Renato stopped her before she could do any real harm. She understandably was upset, screaming all sorts of things at me, begging for me to save her son's father. I couldn't pay attention to her at that particular time; the other shooting victim may have had a better chance of survival. The father of the girl's son didn't seem to have a chance. I had a backup rescue enroute; the worse patient would get priority. I made my way back to the rear bedroom. A young black man lay on his back with a penny sized hole in the middle of his forehead. His eyes were open but never saw me shake my head and walk away. I walked back through the smoky hallway, gun smoke clogging my nostrils toward the dying man in the wingback, put him on the stretcher and wheeled him out the door through the narrow dimly lit hallway and into the rescue, Renato kept us safe until the police gained control of the scene. The guys from engine 12, Renato and me transported him to Rhode Island Hospital Trauma Room, his girlfriend held for questioning. En-route to the hospital I ran an EKG, Renato started a line with a 16 gage catheter and the guys from engine 12 bagged him. Once at the ER, the trauma team cut off his clothes. When his chest was bared, next to a smoking, bleeding hole under his right nipple the image of a barrel of a 44 magnum aimed forward with the inscription, "Thug Life" tattooed below pointed at the doctors trying to save his life. How appropriate.

A party had been in full swing at the apartment prior to the shooting. Some bad blood existed between the partygoers and some kids that wanted to crash. One of the kids who wanted to join the party opened fire, mortally injuring the older brother of a kid who had been murdered only a month before. He was fourteen; gunned down in a playground outside the housing project he called home. The guy bleeding to death in the armchair returned fire, hitting the original shooter in the back. He managed to flee the scene, hole in his back and all. While we were at Rhode Island hospital bringing our victim to the trauma room, a car pulled across the street into the Hasbro Emergency Room parking lot and dumped off a guy who was shot in the back. Were the shootings related? You tell me. The victims "didn't know nothing."

My patient, the one with thug life tattooed to his chest survived his wounds. The guy he shot in the back lived also. The brother of the dead fourteen year old joined his sibling in the graveyard. Days later, people wearing t-shirts bearing pictures of the dead boys were seen on the streets of the hood. "RIP" read the inscriptions below the images. "You will be missed." Too bad the bullets didn't miss them as much as their friends and family will.

ELEVEN

"How did you learn to speak Spanish so well?" I asked Renato as we rode through the city on our war back to Branch Avenue. "Learning Spanish was easy," he explained. "English was the tough part. My Mama and Papi came here from Ecuador in the sixties. All they knew was Spanish. They learned English the best they could and taught us what they knew. Now, me and my brother teach them."

"I didn't know you were Hispanic," I said. "I'm not. I'm Americano!" he said with a contagious laugh. The ride back to the station went quickly. We listened to the local rap station. I found I actually liked the music. "If we're going to work in the hood," Renato explained when he saw me tapping my foot on the dashboard along with "Fitty Cent," "we may as well enjoy the soundtrack!"

The sights and sounds of the shootout lingered in my mind for a little while, and then were replaced with more important things. The images are traumatic; nobody can witness things like that and not be affected to some degree. Years from now, perhaps sooner the emotional carnage could come out of the closet when least expected.

My family was at home, waiting for me to join them as we prepared for Danielle's wedding. Brittany had just graduated college and was actively seeking decent employment. I am fiercely proud of my family and can't imagine ever seeing pictures of their dead faces on a t-shirt saying, "you will be missed." I faced my share of adversity in the seventies and eighties, even spent some time behind bars. There are choices to be made as you reach the crossroads to adulthood. Working for minimum wage isn't nearly as glorious as dealing drugs, or stealing cars, and certainly not as lucrative, but it sets a foundation to build on. Time progresses, opportunities arise and a record of responsibility is established. Without it your choices are limited, and you may end up with a bullet in your head. Nobody gave me the job of Rescue Lieutenant; I earned it through years of hard work, building on my reputation as a dependable member of society. Mistakes were made and learned from. Renato has two boys of his own and a past that I'm sure he would rather have not experienced. He too learned from his mistakes and is well on his way to a respectable career, raising responsible and law-abiding kids. I'm sure they will make their share of stupid mistakes, but their foundation of decency is set by their fathers resolve. His boys are playing sports and studying hard and have every opportunity to be contributing members of society. Choices are made every day by people, hard choices that determine the outcome of future generations. Renato and me grew up on the same streets as the gangs of today, faced the same temptations and found our share of trouble. Maybe our parents loved us more than the kids that were just loaded into our rescue and the medical examiners truck. Maybe they did everything right and circumstances beyond their control decided their fate. Maybe the dead boy's parents don't know any better and are waiting for government programs to keep their kids out of the morgue. For them, the wait is over. I hope others stop waiting and get off their asses and teach their kids a thing or two about respect and responsibility.

One of the good things about the Branch Avenue station is the camaraderie. Twelve firefighters are stationed there at all times. A big house is always more active than a single company house, more people, more fun. Cooking for that many people every day is a challenge. As time spent together progresses tastes become apparent. One guy doesn't like corn, another can't have sugar, and somebody is always on a diet. Somehow it all comes together at mealtime. The complaining is legendary; you can never keep everybody happy. Throughout the ball busting one fact remains; a good cook is welcome in any firehouse. Before becoming a firefighter I worked in kitchens. I spent my high school years washing dishes, and then worked my way up to line and prep cooking in some of Rhode Island's best restaurants. I learned a trick or two in that time and used my knowledge in my new profession much to the delight of the guys. At times my creative side got the best of me and I would prepare some well- intentioned bombs; things like sweet and sour crab stuffed peppers, but for the most part I kept it simple. Individual meat loaf stuffed with spinach, mushrooms and cheese was always a big hit. Linguini with clam sauce went over well on Fridays. I always went all out when I made that dish. I would either dig fresh little necks from the bay if I had time or buy them from the local fish market. Cleaning the shells meticulously, and then adding them to the sauce steams them open from the heat. The fresh juice blends in with the sauce giving it a great taste. Pour the sauce onto a bed of linguini, garnish with the little necks, put a little garlic bread on the side and you have a meal fit for a king - or a firefighter.

Tonight the fare was simple; chowder with homemade stuffies. I was so hungry I could have eaten the shells.

This time of the year there is something for everybody when it comes to sports. The Bruins were my first choice; they were playing the Canadians in the first round of the Stanley Cup Playoffs. The Red Sox had just started their season; no doubt the start of more heartbreak. One guy manned the remote as we ate, switching back and forth from the Bruins to the Red Sox, occasionally foraging into other channels but not for long. Nobody complained about the changing channels, we switch gears with the channel changer. I was banned from the remote years ago; I flicked too fast and stopped at the wrong places. The general rule for stopping the channel surfing is 1, Fire, 2, Explosions, 3, Space Suits, 4, Nudity. 5, Sports. Stopping anywhere else is grounds for remote dismissal.

2056 hrs. (8:56 p.m.)

"Rescue 3 a still alarm."

I shoveled the last spoonful of chowder in my mouth and grabbed a stuffie to go. Renato, not usually assigned to rescue mistakenly believed that he had all of the time in the world to eat. He was still waxing his car while we started eating and had barely taken a bite.

"Rescue 3 respond to the Charlesgate Apartments for a suicidal male."

We left the Branch Avenue Station and headed toward downtown. The Charlesgate Apartments are another Hi-Rise. Elderly residents are still the majority here, but younger disabled people are quickly filling the apartments. When drug and alcohol addiction became an official "disability" a lot of younger people flocked to these places. Some mentally ill and drug addicted people prey on the lonely elderly population. It is a program designed to help that has gone horribly wrong. I didn't know what we would find at our destination, but experience has shown me that a lot of these calls are actually for drug addicted patients who have run out of drugs and money and are looking to "get clean." It is a desperate cry for help made by desperate people.

We arrived on scene, put the rescue in the assigned place and headed for the elevator. Charlesgate is a very clean and well-run Hi-rise. The people who live here don't put up with a lot of nonsense from residents who act out. A few elderly residents were milling about on the first floor, eager to see who called us. We are entertainment for some of these folks who don't get out too much.

The elevator took us to the fifth of fourteen floors, then to the last room on the right hand side of the corridor. "Providence Fire." I say loudly and knock on the door. I stayed to the side in case the patient started blasting the door with a gun. It was a little dramatic, but you never know.

"It's open," came a response from inside.

I opened the door; bright lights, the smell of Lysol disinfectant and a middle-aged man sitting on a folding chair in the middle of an immaculate apartment greeted me. The tile floor was spotless, there was only the chair and a TV in the living room, and the kitchen was empty. There was no evidence of food or cooking supplies. The patient sat in the middle of the living room, dressed in a cotton workout suit with a New England Patriots logo on the front of his sweatshirt. He was slightly overweight and sobbing uncontrollably.

"What's your name?"

"Dennis."

"What the matter?" I asked as Renato quietly looked on.

"I'm being treated for depression but I'm not taking my meds."

"Why not?"

"I ran out." He continued between sobs.

"Why don't you get some more?" I asked.

"I just want to die. I'm sick of fighting it."

He meant it. Whether he planned on killing himself tonight or some time in the near future, I knew that without some serious help this guy would go through with his plan. I have seen too many suicides to not take this threat seriously.

Every time I enter an unfamiliar basement I feel gooseflesh rise from my skin, images of hangings invading my subconscious mind uninvited. One beautiful Saturday morning early in my career a guy in his twenties tied an electrical cord around a nail embedded in a rafter in the basement of the apartment he rented, then strung it around his neck. The ceiling was only six and a half feet high. To die, the man had to use his body weight to strangle himself. Pretty committed.

Three apartments filled the upper floors. The third floor tenant went downstairs to switch her laundry. There she saw her friend from the second floor hanging around the basement. She talked to him for a few minutes while moving her delicates from the washer to the dryer. When she completed her task and walked by her friend toward the stairs she noticed the cord tied around his neck. Only then did she realize he wasn't participating in the conversation. She ran screaming into the street where somebody saw her and called 911. I was there with the crew of Engine 9 in forty-five seconds to see a hysterical girl sobbing uncontrollably in the front of her apartment building. Being the junior man at the time, I was first to enter the basement. A solitary light bulb suspended by a cord swung left and right illuminating the dank basement with dull light, cobwebs and shadows outlining a still form hanging in the corner. Slowly I crept toward him. As I drew closer I noticed his fresh haircut and the tribal tattoo on the back of his neck. His jeans were sagging, at least six inches touching the dirty cement floor. I shook him, turned him toward me. I saw the extension cord tied tightly around his neck and the glazed look in his eyes, still open, and then felt his skin as cold as midnight in January. I was standing in a puddle of piss, his, not mine, but couldn't move, frozen in place by the horror I witnessed. His skin was a greenish gray, a perfect match to the worn army fatigue jacket he wore. Finally the trance was broken and I stumbled up the creaking stairs into the bright sunlight. The girl who found him had gained control of herself by now and was sitting with a bunch of twenty-something year olds who had huddled by the basement window, crouching to get a better look through the dusty glass. "I knew he was going to do it!" one of the kids exclaimed, barely able to conceal his excitement. "He said he was going to do it, boy did he! I thought he'd pussy out and OD. Man, he did it right!" he said, worshiping his hero, now hanging dead in the basement. Days later I read the boy's obituary. He was a talented tattoo artist with a loving family from Smithfield, RI. He played hockey in high school and loved to write. He moved to Wickenden Street on the east side and got involved with a notorious group of junkies. No second chance for him.

I don't understand what goes wrong with some people. I'm sure Dennis was not sitting here sobbing and wanting to die purposely and was nothing like the thrill seeking junkies on Wickenden Street. He appeared like any other guy in his forties, more at home in a bar having a beer with his friends and watching the game than sitting by himself in a sparse and immaculate apartment crying. I saw posters and championship banners from the Patriots, Red Sox and Bruins on the walls and tried to engage in some sports talk, but he wouldn't bite. He sobbed as we walked him out to the truck and transported him to Rhode Island Hospital. There he was put under observation until a Psychologist had time to assess him, then he would be referred for outpatient counseling, or committed to a Psychiatric hospital. The fact that he called 911 for help was encouraging; I hope that he gets some help before it is too late.

I had planned on listening to the end of the Bruins game on the radio as we made our way back to the station, but I had lost interest.

TWELVE

Half way back to the Branch Avenue fire station fire alarm dispatched Engine 14 to the intersection of Atwells Avenue and Harris for a motor vehicle accident. All of the Providence rescues were out on calls. I was going at a pretty good pace and I needed a break. A typical rescue run takes between thirty minutes and an hour depending on the severity of the emergency. Between calls your brain and body catches up. I don't normally feel it, but there is a discernable increase in my stress when I am on duty. It takes a few days off for me to realize that I have been operating on a different level.

My first impulse was to ignore the radio and recuperate. There is no way that five rescues can keep up with the demand, if I didn't respond to this call, another would be right behind it. My conscience took over, if I didn't take this run and there were serious injuries the victims will be the ones who pay. Somebody's mother, lover, friend or child could be involved in the accident in need of medical care. I keyed the mike.

2129 hrs. (9:29 p.m.)

"Rescue 3 to fire Alarm, we are clearing Rhode Island, we'll handle."

"You have it Rescue 3, we have a report of four cars involved."

Renato hit the lights and sirens, reversed direction and headed to the scene. The majority of auto accidents in the city seldom result in life threatening injuries. Minor scrapes and bumps, small lacerations and the like are common. The most prevalent injuries are neck and back pain. Soft tissue injury is also common. Insurance fraud is epidemic. Lawyers advertise their business on daytime TV, their premise being that if somebody caused an accident, that person should pay. Often there is no visible damage to the vehicles or occupants, but in hopes of a big insurance settlement some victims go to the hospital. Talent agents could scout accident scenes looking for the next big star, the acting is remarkable. Some of the injuries are legitimate, most are not.

Four cars, probably ten people involved could tie up the EMS system for hours. If every person on scene claims to be injured, at least five rescues will have to respond. The patients have to be placed on a long back board, a cervical collar applied and transported per state protocol lying on their back and immobilized. The victims must be extricated from the cars, a process that usually takes three firefighters. If you neglect to do the extrication perfectly, you can and will be sued. Lawyers can be unscrupulous. There are actually advertisements asking the public if EMS and Emergency room personnel have mistreated them, and if so, you can "Make Them Pay!"

We navigated through the traffic on Atwells and pulled up to the accident scene. The officer of Engine 14, Bob Dunne had assessed the accident scene and gave me his report.

"Minor damage all around, looks like everybody's refusing."

"That's a miracle," I said.

"We've got an old guy in the white Buick who says his shoulder hurts, you might want to get him to sign a refusal."

"Good idea, thanks Bob."

The four cars that were involved in the accident had all pulled over to the side of the road, except for the white Buick. I walked over to the driver's side and saw a well-dressed man in his eighties sitting at the wheel.

"Sir, are you hurt?" I asked.

"Yup," he answered, looking strait ahead.

"Where are you hurt?"

"My shoulder, I'm waiting for my wife," he replied.

"If you want to be seen at the hospital, we'll take you, your wife can meet us there."

"I'm not doing anything without my wife," he said, all business.

"That's fine, but you're tying up traffic. Why don't you let us move your car out of the way until your wife gets here?" I tried.

"Nope."

"Then sign this refusal and wait for the police. I can't wait here all night."

"I don't care what you do, I'm not refusing, and I'm not signing anything. I'm waiting for my wife." This guy was really starting to get on my nerves.

"We're not waiting for your wife, so come with us or sign the refusal."

"When my wife gets here I'll decide what to do," he says, and that appears to be the end of it, for him anyway.

"When is your wife getting here?" I asked. "When she gets here," he replied.

The man refused treatment, refused to sign the refusal form and refused to move his car from the intersection. Anybody that refuses treatment is required to sign a refusal if they are competent. The man in the Buick is competent; he is just an asshole. The police had not made it to the scene yet, the guy could sit in the intersection for the rest of his life for all that I cared. I walked away from the car, unsigned report in my hand and back to Lt. Dunne.

"Bob, the guy in the Buick won't come with us, won't move his car and won't do anything until his wife gets here."

"Don't worry about it," Bob says, "we'll wait here for the police. Not much you can do with a guy like that. Try to get some rest."

Lieutenant Dunne has been with the fire department for at least twenty years. He is one of the last of a dying breed. He has done it all. He loves the job and is one of the most liked and respected people we have. Firefighters are not given respect just because they are firefighters. The respect is earned on the streets and in the stations. Bob has earned the respect that he now enjoys by being a hard-nosed front-line firefighter as well as a great guy in the station. He respects the guys working the rescues and understands our workload is extreme. He would give you the shirt off of his back in a blizzard if you needed it, I'd do the same for him. His willingness to stay on scene gave us the opportunity to get back to the station and rest for a little while, and lets Renato finish his dinner.

Renato had assessed the other passengers in the cars involved and confirmed that there were no injuries. I shook Bob's hand and we left the scene. I explained to Renato during to ride back to the station what had happened. Without trying, Bob had earned the respect of another new guy. The kids striving to make their mark as firefighters never forget little gestures from grizzled veterans.

The trip back down Atwells Avenue toward home was a little more peaceful. Bob had bought us a little time. The restaurants and clubs were in full swing. There were plenty of sights to see as we trawled down the busy street. The restaurants lining the street are beyond compare, the cuisine and atmosphere unparalleled, spoiling the residents in the area. Only when traveling away from the city do we realize the treasure we have in our own backyard.

We heard on the radio that both the Red Sox and Bruins won their games. I wished that Dennis could have shared my happiness rather than sitting at RI Hospital under a suicide watch waiting for a psych evaluation. Renato it turned out is a Yankee fan. Too bad. I had hoped to lure him into the rescue division as a possible replacement for Mike, but realized that would not be possible. Yankee fans have genetic defects making it impossible for them to behave like civilized human beings.

It was nearly ten o'clock. If I had any luck I would make it back to the station, call my wife and get some rest. It had been an exhausting day, but not one without a few high points. Every run doesn't end with the satisfaction of making a difference in somebody's life, a lot of our calls are routine transports, but if you can squeeze one or two good ones in during the course of a day it makes the mundane worthwhile. I try to keep that in mind as the long shift grinds on. The difficult, life-threatening responses are easy to handle; instinct and training guides you. Routine calls to us are emergencies to the people making the calls. Some are looking for a ride, but a majority of the callers truly believe that their situation warrants a fire department response. By treating each caller with respect I have learned to respect myself.

THIRTEEN

Back at the Branch Avenue station the dinner dishes had been cleared, the remains of Renato's meal were covered with tin foil and set aside and the guys were either playing cards or in the dormitory getting some rest. I went to my office to call Cheryl and hopefully get a little sleep. My cell phone was almost dead, enough juice for one more call. I dialed the number and hit send.

"Hello," she answered on the first ring.

"Hi babe, it's me."

"Who else would it be at ten-thirty?"

"Your boyfriend."

"He already came and left."

"I hope he didn't wear you out, I'll be home tomorrow."

"I think I'll be too tired."

"You're never too tired for me."

"Yeah right, how is your night?"

"Not bad, we had chowder and stuffies."

"How are you holding up?"

"Pretty good, I'm going to get a little rest, I'll call you in the morning."

The overhead lights clicked on and the PA system came to life. I made a silent prayer to the rescue Gods that the engine or ladder was going. My prayers went unanswered.

"Rescue 3 a still alarm"

"So much for the rest, I've got a run."
"Be careful."
"Of course, love you, bye.
"Love you too."

2233 hrs. (10:33 p.m.)

"Rescue 3, respond to 3 Hagan Street at the Hagan Manor for a man who wants his testicles looked at." The dispatcher barely concealed his amusement. The couch looked so inviting, but duty called.

"Rescue 3, responding."

My cell phone rang as I slid the pole. I knew it was Cheryl. She sometimes listens to a scanner that we have at the house. She usually shuts it off at bedtime and probably had her fingers on the off knob when this call came in.

"Hello"
"Did I just hear that you are going to look at somebody's testicles?"
"That's right, I am an expert, and I have a few of my own you know."
"Try not to touch them."
"Very funny." I heard her chuckling as I hit the end button on the cell phone.

"Do we really have to look at somebody's testicles?" asked Renato on the way to Hagan Manor.

"We don't have to, the junior man has to," I said with a grin. "Rank has its privileges."

""What if somebody wanted their breasts looked at?" Renato asked.

"I'd have to assess the situation before making that decision," I answered.

"All my life I wanted to be a firefighter. I just didn't know testicle tests were part of the job," said Renato with resignation. He will do whatever it takes, I can tell he is that kind of guy.

The ride from the station to Hagan Manor took about five minutes. The place is a three level apartment building full of elderly and disabled people. There are not too many troublemakers here, mostly older folks. Whenever I have been called here there has always been a welcoming committee at the door telling us who called and what for. Somebody usually accompanies us to the person's room. Living there is good if you don't mind people knowing your business. They do seem to take care of each other.

We pulled in front of the building, got the stretcher off of the truck just in case and headed for the door. The housecoat brigade greeted us. The brigade can be found at every elderly housing complex in the city. Day and night they patrol the corridors, never sleeping, always alert. Three women dressed in colorful housecoats waited to help us in the door and to the elevator. They somehow knew what were here for; the delight on their faces barely concealed. This one will be talked about for weeks, maybe even months.

We ditched the ladies, much to their chagrin and no easy task and headed for the victim's door. He was inside, waiting.

"What's the problem?" I asked once we were in with the door closed.

"My testicles are swollen. Look at them; they're the size of cantaloupes." He lowers his sweatpants to expose his testicles which are indeed the size of cantaloupes. "It's not the first time. I have a heart condition that causes lower extremity swelling. My balls are the first things to grow"

"How long has this been going on?"

"Just about two days. My doctor is at Miriam, I need to get there."

"We'll take you but this isn't an emergency," I said. "In the future you should either arrange transportation or call a private ambulance. We only have five trucks and can't be tied up on routine medical transports." I explained the situation to the patient but he could care less. He called 911 for transport, and truly believed that we were required to cater to his wishes. Renato and I can barely contain ourselves, but somehow pull it off and act like professionals.

Miriam hospital is one of seven area hospitals that we transport to. We are only required to transport to the nearest hospital, but can make exceptions. Roger Williams Medical Center is closer to us, but I decided to be a sport and take this guy to Miriam. The patient can't walk without rubbing his testicles, so we put him on the stretcher and wheeled him to the truck. The housecoat brigade waited at the door to send us off.

Once in the truck Renato got the patient's vital signs and I asked the necessary questions. He was only fifty years old. Three years ago he was diagnosed with a heart problem and his life had gone downhill since. His wife left him; he lost his job and was living on disability. He had only lived at the Hagan Manor for three months but said he was starting to feel good about things again. The people there were a little nosy, but at least they cared.

Miriam hospital is located on the East Side. I hadn't been there in some time. They are affiliated with Rhode Island Hospital and the same doctors practice at both facilities.

The temptation to treat this patient in a lighthearted manner was overwhelming. I couldn't resist having a little fun with Christy, who was working triage.

"Fifty year old male, conscious and alert, vitals stable." I said. Christy didn't look up from her report, just wrote down what I told her. I continued my report in a deadpan voice as if reading an excerpt from biology textbook. "Testicles the size of cantaloupes, otherwise everything appears normal." That got a rise out of her. The look on her face was priceless. The patient wasn't pleased but that's what he got for calling 911 for a free ride to the hospital.

Christy, a naturally beautiful nurse with spectacular blue eyes that seem to see right through me was working the triage desk on my first night in charge of a rescue. I was scared to death; the responsibility on rescue can be overwhelming when new and inexperienced. I was bringing a patient to her suffering from difficulty breathing. While giving my report on the patient's condition in what I believed to be a very professional and efficient manner I mentioned that the patients Pulsox reading was only ninety-one %. Christy looked me in the eye and asked if the reading was 'on room air,' a very common reference determining if the patient was using supplemental oxygen. In my mind, I heard her say 'on rumeir' and thought that she was flirting with me by speaking French. I responded with a big grin, and said, "Oui, oui." She gave me a wry look and asked again, "on room air?" I was totally embarrassed; she shook her head and walked away. I've never lived it down though she claims to not remember the incident at all. I think she's being kind.

Our patient was checked in, his cantaloupes being tended to and the paperwork done. I was hoping for a quiet night. e rolled out of the ambulance bay at Miriam down the hilly road toward home.

FOURTEEN

"Rescue 3 a still alarm."

The blow lights woke me before the PA system came to life. I looked at my watch through blurry eyes and was shocked to find that I had been unconscious for ten minutes. It felt like hours. When a call comes in to the Fire Alarm office, the dispatchers, after sorting out the information from the caller hit a switch on their console beginning the process of dispatching the proper response. On our end, the first indication that we are going out is the activation of the "blow lights." Every overhead light in the building is wired directly to the fire alarm office, when they trip the switch the building goes from serene darkness to intense daylight. A few years of experience equips you with a sixth sense, a low hum, only able to be heard by some species of canine and rescue veterans fills the air before the light blinds you. I felt the lights before they came on.

0004 hrs. (12:04 a.m.)

"Rescue 3, respond to 8 Stimson Street for a man bleeding from the head." I keyed my portable; I never had the chance to take it off of my belt.

"Rescue 3 on the way.

I rested for a minute on the bunk trying to figure out if this was a dream or reality. Just in case I wasn't dreaming, I slipped on my shoes and headed for the truck. Renato was already there, the motor running.

"I know where that is!" Renato exclaims. "My brother used to live over there. We'll be there in no time!" I am refreshed by his enthusiasm. There is nothing worse than a miserable partner. With Mike leaving I'm worried about my future on the rescue truck. Renato seems to be a great guy, but most young guys want nothing to do with rescue. The thrill of firefighting is understandably something that takes all of the good guys away from EMS.

We rode to the call in silence. I silently asked myself why I do this. The money is better, but the real reason is because I am one of the fortunate few who can say he loves his job. For ten years I worked the engine and ladder trucks. I fought a lot of fires in that time and learned a lot. The adrenaline rush felt while driving toward a fully involved house fire in the middle of the night, past people running away from the inferno's with what belongings they could gather carried on their backs is indescribable. The pungent smell of smoke gets heavier the closer you get. Running into a burning building that anybody with a rational mind would be running out of is something that firefighters live for. I've spotted ladder trucks next to burning buildings, extended aerial ladders and rescued people hanging out of windows. On cold, wintry nights on rooftops full of ice I've clung to precipices, straddled peaks and chopped holes to ventilate. I've forced open doors, or knocked them down and attacked fires from the inside. I've dragged inch and ¾ hoselines equipped with a Task Force Tips capable of discharging 50-350 gallons of water per minute through smoke filled buildings. I've felt the heat, then found the fire; it's destructive power raging unchallenged and unstoppable, gaining strength; until it met me. I've given the order, "turn in my line!" as flames rolled toward me and overhead, threatening to flash over, waiting for the pump operator to open the gate in time to release 90 pounds of pressurized water to the end of my line. I've knocked the fires down and waited for the smoke to clear. I couldn't imagine doing anything else.

Then, I was transferred to the rescue division. I was only supposed to go for six months. I found out that I wanted to stay. Had I not spent ten years on the front line firefighting trucks, I never would have been able to change my career path. I still miss the smoke and fire, and some day might go back. For now, EMS is my life. It is more suited to my personality anyway. Thinking back to my childhood and the dreams I had, it was the obvious choice.

The popular television show *Emergency* was my favorite show back in the seventies. Johnny Gage and Roy Desoto were my first role models. As early as I can remember, I wanted to do this kind of work. When we played war games as kids I always wanted to be the medic. My vision of wartime heroism never involved killing the enemy, rather I dreamed of running through the rice paddies in Cambodia, bullets whizzing past my head, close enough to smell gunpowder, mortar rounds exploding all around me with dead guys everywhere. Disregarding my own safety I would go to the aid of my fallen comrades, taking bullets along the way, spitting out shrapnel and pushing morphine into the wounded soldiers. Once I killed their pain, I would carry the fallen on my back, using the fireman's carry, back to the jungle and the safety of my unit. "Thanks Doc," was all that I needed to hear.

"Rescue 3 on the scene." I said into the mike.

Engine 9 was already there. The victim was being helped down the front steps of his apartment house, a firefighter on each side, holding him up. I saw inside the house Arabic writing on posters adorning the walls.

He had a towel on top on his head, covered in blood. It dripped from the edges, onto his silk shirt and sidewalk.

The officer of Engine 9 gave me his report.

"Thirty-four old male, smashed his head on a stone table, no loss of consciousness, but he has a huge laceration to the top of his head."

"I can see that." I said.

The patient walked into the truck, holding the bloody towel on his head and sat in my seat, dripping blood everywhere.

"You're sitting in my seat," I told him, trying to mask my irritation.

"I don't care, my head is splitting." He said with a middle-eastern accent.

"Get out of my seat." I told him and pointed to the bench next to the stretcher. He reluctantly moved, mumbling something, I didn't care what.

It had been three years since 9-11 but the wounds still ran deep. I was not proud of the fact that I looked at this patient with disdain. I'm sure he had nothing whatsoever to do with the terrorist attacks on that day, but something residing deep within me came to the surface and it took every ounce of restraint for me to treat him with the respect I knew he deserved. I have always prided myself on my fairness and respect for people of all races, religions and sexual preferences. I don't want to think poorly of this man, bleeding profusely from a serious wound to the top of his head, but I can't stop it. It bothers me that I can't see him as just another person who needs help. Something snapped in me on that beautiful September day and I pray that I am not broken forever.

I have worn the turnout gear, Scott pack strapped to my back and carried the irons and hi-rise packs up numerous flights of stairs to fight fires on the upper floors of tall office buildings. I have felt the exhaustion from carrying equipment up flight after flight of stairs, wondering if you would have anything left when you finally got to the fire. Thankfully, I never felt what those New York City firefighters felt as they walked bravely up those stairs into heaven. Their sacrifice doesn't fill me with pride in my profession, it fills me with rage at the people who perpetrated that heinous crime, and continue to do so in the name of Allah. God damn them all.

That attitude wasn't going to help the guy in my rescue. I'm slowly becoming more rational when it comes to dealing with people from the Middle East. I truly don't want the rage to live inside me any more.

The back of the rescue is very confined. Here, I am the alpha-male. I need my space to be unspoiled. It's not a lot to ask, one small corner in the back. I hate for it to be contaminated. This guy was off to a bad start. I sprayed my seat with disinfectant and wiped it with a clean towel before I sat and begin figuring out what is going on.

"What happened?" I asked.

"I tripped on a rug that I had rolled up in the corner of my kitchen. Before I could get my balance, I fell into the table. I hit my head, I'm losing a lot of blood."

"I can see that. Renato, get a board." I reached into the overhead compartment and got a cervical collar. The device was collapsible; I had to make some adjustments before applying it to the patient. Before I did that I took a look at the injury. Lifting the towel from the man's head I saw an enormous laceration, at least twelve inches circling the top of his head. I couldn't believe that he wasn't knocked out cold. I wasn't mad at him anymore.

"I can't believe you weren't knocked out cold!" I said to him as I put the collar around his neck. Renato had come to the back door with a long backboard. I took it from him and put it on the stretcher.

"Here, sit here," I said pointing to the middle of the purple, hard plastic board. He did as I asked. I dressed his wound with a trauma dressing, wrapped his head with some gauze and helped him lay onto his back. It is a little uncomfortable at first, and then becomes unbearable. I lied to him as he grimaced.

"You will get used to the backboard. It only hurts for a little while."

Renato got his blood pressure and pulse, while I checked his pupils and asked him a few questions.

"Do you know what day it is?"

"It is Thursday morning, the 8th of April at 12:30 in the morning." he responded. He was more alert than me, I realized as I looked into his pupils and saw that they were equal in size and reactive to light. I started an IV because Renato has informed me that his pulse was 124, his Blood pressure 130/90. The blood pressure was fine, his pulse irregular. A rapid pulse is indicative of a potentially serious head injury. I placed a non-re-breather over his mouth and nose after setting the flow to 10 liters.

I handed Renato the EKG leads.

"White right, smoke over fire," he said with a smile, reciting the age-old way to remember where on the body to place the EKG leads. The monitor's green light glowed and showed a sinus rhythm, rapidly moving along. I noted "sinus tach" on the state report and recorded the other vital signs.

"You guys are all set," I said to the members of Engine 9 who had been outside of the truck waiting to see if they could be of assistance. If the situation warranted, I would have needed one of their guys in the back with us to help with the patient and another of them to drive the rescue. This patient was stable. The engine went back in service and we went to Rhode Island Hospital. The patient's wife had locked up the house and rode in the back of the rescue with us, holding her husband's hand during transport. I found out that they were from India. He was a professor at Brown University and she was a student. They were two young professionals in love hoping to start a life in the United States in the medical field, helping others. Damn those terrorists for turning me into a cynical bastard.

Things at the hospital were crazy. Elliot, a gentle giant security guard from Alabama was waiting outside the ER doors. He looked at our patient and shook his head. Dressed in his security uniform and well over six feet tall and weighing two fifty at least he makes an intimidating presence. It is unfortunate that the hospital has to hire security guards, but the city is a nut house, and all of the nuts think this is their home.

We moved our patient from our stretcher onto the hospital bed and wheeled him in. Tonya was at the triage desk, waiting for my report.

"What do you have?" she asked, no nonsense in her demeanor. I was not fooled. She is a riot when given the chance. Nobody is better when the pressure is on; though she tolerates incompetence with barely concealed contempt. We have been through this hundreds of times and have learned to trust each other. I gave the report; she assessed the patient, agreed with my findings and started the procedure of his care. This patient was going to the trauma room because of his unstable vital signs. Renato had cleaned and restocked the truck, ready for the next patient as we wheeled back into the city.

FIFTEEN

We had made it back to the station. Renato still hadn't finished his dinner. It takes a while to learn to eat at rescue speed.

"If it wasn't so busy, I wouldn't mind staying on Rescue for a while," he said while shoveling cold stuffies into his mouth and dribbling clam chowder down his chin. "It's a great way to learn the streets. I'll lose some weight too if I never get a chance to eat," he laughed.

"In six months on rescue I learned more streets than ten years on the trucks. It's different over here. You have a little more time to figure out where you are going. When a call comes in for a fire, you had better know where it is without thinking. There's nothing worse than blowing a street and having a ladder truck and chief follow you down the wrong road," I told him, leaving out the fact that it happened to me, more than once.

"Has that happened?" he asked.

"More than once." I replied, hiding my grin by looking out the side window.

"Rescue 5 and Engine 2 a still alarm."

"You have got to be kidding," said Renato as I keyed the mike.

"Rescue 3 in service." I said.

"Roger, Rescue 3, Rescue 5 you can disregard. Rescue 3 and Engine 2, respond to Route 95 North at exit 24 for an MVA."

The stuffies and chowder disappeared as we walked down the stairs toward the apparatus. Renato started the engine, hit the lights and siren and we were on our way.

0107 hrs. (1:07 a.m.)

A highway response has its own set of potential problems. Scene safety is paramount. Every year firefighters and police officers are killed on the highways, struck by cars. At this time of night, the possibility of a drunk driver passing the emergency scene is great. I always tell my drivers who are new on the truck the same thing.

"Be careful, these people WILL kill you."

"I know, we got hit on Engine 2 last week." Renato says. "Some drunk slammed into the back of the truck, then took off. The funny thing was, his license plate got embedded in the trucks bumper."

"Bad luck for him," I said. Sometimes the good guys get a break.

Engine 2 had arrived on scene and transmitted their findings.

"Engine 2 to fire alarm, we have a twenty-five year old male, conscious and alert complaining of neck and back pain, a laceration to his forehead."

"Rescue 1 received." I said into the truck microphone as we continued to the accident scene on 95 North. Traffic was light, the roads were dry, visibility was good and there was only one victim. Chances were good that a drunk driver waited for us further up the road.

"Rescue 1 on the scene." Engine 2 had blocked the two low speed travel lanes by parking their truck across the lanes with their emergency lights activated. The State Police were on the scene, directly in front of the engine. A four-door sedan was stopped in front of the State Police vehicle, it's nose imbedded in a guardrail.

The air bags had deployed and the windshield was broken. I couldn't tell if the air bag broke the windshield or the driver's head. I planned on giving him a thorough going over when I got him in the truck. I had seen hundreds of similar scenes over the years. The driver was standing next to the police officer, his arms waving around as he proclaimed his innocence. Without being in earshot, I knew what he is saying.

"I was doing the speed limit and minding my own business. A big truck came out of nowhere and cut me off. He rode me right into the guardrail and kept on going. I only had a few beers."

We stopped the rescue in front of the victim's car and walked over to him, passersby flying past looked at us instead of the road.

"What's his story?" I asked the trooper

"He says he was cut off by a trucker who kept on going."

"Has he been drinking?" I asked.

"A couple of beers," says the trooper with a knowing smile.

"Are you hurt?" I asked the victim. He looked off into space.

"Hey buddy, are you hurt?" I asked again, this time taking his arm and shaking him as I spoke.

"I think so," he responded.

"What do you mean, you think so. Are you or aren't you?"

"I think so."

"Get in the truck." I said with resignation. This guy looked wasted, but there is always the possibility of a head injury causing his lethargic reaction to my questions. We brought him to the back of the truck. Renato had gotten another long board from the side compartment and we got him ready for transport. He complained about everything; the blood pressure cuff was too tight, the cervical collar hurt, the backboard was too hard and on and on. The State Trooper came to the back of the rescue to give him a ticket, then the complaining really started. His car was be towed to a garage where it was stored until he could retrieve it. Engine 2 waited until we cleared the highway, providing safety.

Renato got in front to drive and I finished in the back. The patient didn't give me any more information, but I had gotten all that I needed from the trooper. His vital signs were perfect, blood pressure 120/70, his pulse 68. He had a one-inch superficial laceration above his right eye. His eyes were bloodshot, and he smelled of booze. I put this information on the state report. Whether or not he was charged with drunk driving was up to the police. I hoped he was charged. This guy could have killed somebody instead of ruining a perfectly good guardrail.

Renato took the next exit from 95 north, made a quick turnaround in Pawtucket and got back on 95 heading south toward Rhode Island Hospital. My patient layed quietly on the backboard, his neck immobilized by the cervical collar and looked up at the ceiling. I looked out the back windows of the rig, watching Providence glide by backwards.

I hoped the city slept until daybreak, I needed the rest. Sometimes the rescue gods are kind, more often they are not. We made our way back to quarters, Renato to the dorm, myself to my office. I was sleeping within seconds, I'm sure Renato was too.

SIXTEEN

"Rescue 3 a still alarm."

0230 hrs. (2:30 a.m.)

It felt like I had been sleeping for hours when the lights came on and the speaker started to blare. The first words were indecipherable; luckily the dispatchers repeat the address a few times.

"Rescue 3 respond with Engine 15 to 174 Putnam street for an emotional woman with a knife, bleeding from the wrists."

Great. Just what I needed. My forty-three year old body felt sixty-five as I stood, the pain in my creaky knees making its way up my back and into my shoulders. My joints groaned as I put my rebellious body back into action. An hour's sleep is a great nap, but no substitute for a nights sleep. Renato waited in the truck as I struggled down the stairs and into the rig.

Putnam Street is located in the Olneyville section of the city, about a mile down the road from Atwells Avenue and Federal Hill. The neighborhood got its name from Christopher Olney, who in 1785 operated a gristmill and paper mill there. Before that, Native Americans lived there and called their settlement Woonasquatucket," meaning "at the head of the tidewater." In the 19th century the area was one of the leading industrial centers in the country. After WWII textiles became the driving force of Olneyville's economy. Workers lived in two or three family homes nearby. As the textile industry moved to the southern states the jewelry industry took over. There were not enough good jobs to go around and the population declined. The area was notorious in the late sixties and seventies as poverty and crime invaded the area. It still has a way to go, but recent improvements in the area have made it an attractive destination for immigrant families.

Engine 15 was with the police at our destination. The fifteens officer gave his report by radio, "Engine 15 to Rescue 3, we have a forty six year old female, conscious and alert but suffering from delusions, minor lacerations to the top of her wrists."

"Rescue 3 received."

"What are delusions?" asked Renato as we approached the house.

"You are about to find out," I answered. I had no idea what to expect.

The patient sat on a wooden chair in the middle of the front room in the first floor apartment. The sheets being used as curtains were tattered and filthy, clothes were strewn around the room. The smell of unwashed laundry and skin invaded my senses as soon as I entered the home.

"What's going on?" I asked the patient. She looked at me without focusing her wild eyes on mine, crouched lower in the chair and said, "Vicky is in charge, ask her."

I looked around the room for another woman but only saw a skinny man sitting on a white couch in the other end of the room. The couch he sat on had the look of a curbside sale.

"Where's Vicky?"

"I'm right here," said the woman.

"Why are your wrists bleeding?"

"Because Doris is bad and I want to hurt her."

"Who's Doris?"

"I put her away."

"Where?"

"Way down inside me where she'll never come back."

It all came together. Doris was either playing a dangerous game with us or she truly had a split personality.

"Can I talk to Doris?" I asked as the three firefighters from Engine 15, four police officers and Renato looked on.

"I'll kill her if she comes back."

"We are going to take you to the hospital so you can get some help," I said. No use pussyfooting around. Any sign of indecision on my part would strengthen her delusions.

"I'm not going to a hospital! Vicky wants to play!"

I had to let her know she had no choice in the matter. I have a weird knack for talking sense into crazy people, probably from talking to myself for years.

"Vicky, you hurt Doris and I have to get her to the hospital. I can't leave her here with you or you might kill her.

"I like to play with knives," she said and stood up. The police officers began to move toward her but I raised my hand and they stopped. They wanted to end this drama as quickly as possible without having to restrain Vicky/Doris. They trusted me and let me go on for a while. Vicky/Doris sat back down and began crying. She wrapped her arms around her knees and rocked gently back and forth as she sobbed. I closed in slowly, attempting to gain her trust. When I was three feet away I stopped, crouched to her level and asked her, "Are you ready to get some help."

"I've got Vicky in bondage. Let's go before she escapes."

That was music to my ears. Doris was back and cooperative. Rhode Island Hospital was only five minutes away.

"Do you want one of my guys to ride with you in case she acts up? Asked Dick, the officer of Engine 15.

"I should be all right, there's only two of them." My answer lifted most of the tension from the room. Even Doris chuckled. The skinny man looked relieved and the police began to retreat. As we walked out the door into the chilly night air Vicky returned.

"I like to play!" said our patient.

"I'll take you up on that offer," I told Dick. Will, one of the guys from Engine 15 accompanied us as we rode through Olneyville, up Atwells Avenue toward Route 95. One of the police cruisers followed us to the hospital. Doris returned once we got rolling, sobbing most of the way. I will never know if the whole thing was an act or if she truly was sick. Psychological disorders such as schizophrenia and bi-polar disorder are relatively common. I had a feeling that Doris was in the manic stage of her bi-polar disorder and playing with us. She had five firefighters, four police officers and her skinny boyfriend catering to her whims for half an hour. Not a bad night's work for the two of them.

All I knew was that if I didn't get a little shut-eye my alter ego would appear. I am not proud of my behavior at times, especially when lack of sleep tries my patience with people who call 911 for a ride to the hospital. It sometimes feels as though I'm being tested by the people of the city who seem to never sleep. We are routinely called between the hours of midnight and six in the morning for sore throats, headaches, toothaches, nightmares, tummy aches, and the like. It comes with the territory, and I knew that before getting onto the rescue truck, but it still drives me crazy. Most of the time I handle the abuse well, but lack of sleep takes my perspective away. Most of the people who call us feel that their emergency is the real deal and I treat them accordingly. There are times, thankfully not too often that the long hours add up and I lash out at the people who have called for help.

The city felt quiet. I looked forward to three hours uninterrupted rest. Renato was full of energy and ran up the twenty four stairs from the apparatus floor to the living quarters two at a time. Youth, wasted on the young. I used the railing to pull my tired, aching body up the stairs toward my office and into the rack.

SEVENTEEN

I feel the speeding truck sway in rhythm with the winding road, the IV bag swinging back and forth with each turn, hypnotic if I choose to be captured by its spell. Moonlight filters through the back windows of the rig illuminating the cramped space. I am alone with a dying patient, his silence haunting, the only sound was his labored breathing which had turned from gasps to a death rattle. I fumbled with the catheter; my hands seeming to hold the needle for the first time. Where is all the help, I wondered as I butchered my patient's arms with pathetic attempts to start a line. For the first time since I was a trainee I felt panic. The lights flickered as the truck started shaking, the speed too much to handle I shouted to the front for the driver to slow down, but nobody answered. The oxygen mask fell from my patient's face, revealing his identity. He looked at me with piercing blue eyes that I remembered so well from my childhood. With surprising strength he grabbed my shirt with both of his hands and pulled me within inches of his face. The smell of beer consumed the tight space between us, another memory stirred.

"You never could do anything right," my father said between dying gasps for air. There is no menace in his tone, just resignation. I felt his disappointment to the depths of my soul. If only I could have saved him

from the cancer that ravaged his body fifteen years ago he would have lived to see that I actually could do something right. I lifted him from the stretcher, shook him and shouted,

"I did it, Dad. I'm going to be all right! I straitened out right after you died!" My words are too late, just as I was too late getting my life together.

He died in my nightmare, just as dead as that night fifteen years ago when he died in my arms, convinced that I was a bum. The driver of the truck turned around. My mother, her face glimmering in the dull moonlight.

"Killed him again," she said as the truck careened out of control.

"Rescue 3 a still alarm."

I was frozen in place, awakened by the familiar tone and covered in sweat, the sheets of my bunk a twisted wreck. My office was mercifully bathed in bright fluorescent light. I looked around and saw I was the only one there. I checked my watch through blurry eyes, 0530. Sometimes it is better not to sleep during long shifts.

0530 hrs. (5:30 a.m.)

"Rescue 3 and Engine 12, respond to 534 Sandringham Avenue for an elderly female with difficulty breathing, history of CHF.

I had responded to this type of emergency dozens of times since coming to rescue. Engine 12's district is full of single-family homes with a large number of elderly residents. Rescue 3 responds to medical emergencies dealing with the elderly more than the other four trucks combined. There are eleven nursing homes or elderly hi-rises in the district, the potential for calls enormous. Providence

College is prominent in the area; the students and faculty mingle with long-term residents.

This time I had to wait for Renato to get to the truck. He made it to the apparatus floor thirty seconds after me, got in and started the engine. Once again the overhead doors opened, this time the first hint of light is evident as darkness grudgingly gave way to dawn. Sunrise was still an hour away, but the start of a new day had begun.

"Do you know where we're going?" I asked.

"Sandringham, it's over by Engine 12." He responded gruffly.

We both had bugs in our heads from lack of sleep. Renato put his brain on automatic pilot and headed toward the Admiral Street fire station and I looked for the street in the directory. Every truck has a street guide, they come in handy. Under normal circumstances, I would have know exactly where the street was located, but my brain wasn't fully awake yet so I needed a little help from the book. The streets were deserted, we kept the sirens off during our ride. It made no sense waking the residents up, the less people awake, the less chances of them calling 911. It was all about self-preservation at this hour.

In the five minutes it took for us to get from Branch Avenue to Sandringham, I became fully awake. Engine 12 relayed the message from the house:

"Engine 12 to Fire Alarm, advise rescue we have an eighty-two year old female, conscious and alert complaining of difficulty breathing, we're getting vital signs now but she is obvious distress. History of CHF.

"Rescue 3 received." The information from Engine 12 helped put my mind in gear. An elderly lady with trouble breathing, in obvious distress and a history of Congestive Heart Failure is a serious situation. Her lungs were filling up with fluid because her left ventricle, the part of the heart responsible for pumping blood through the circulatory system was weak and not able to keep the bodily fluid moving. As a result, her lungs were filling with fluid, her airflow diminished. Her blood pressure was probably skyrocketing and her pulse greatly increasing as her heart tried to compensate for the lack of powerful beats with rapid, weaker ones.

"Engine 12 to Fire Alarm, advise Rescue 3 her BP is 220/115 with a pulse of 120."

"Rescue 3 received, on the scene."

We pulled in front a beautifully kept colonial, the front door open and well lit.

"Get the chair," I told Renato as I made my way into the home. A set of stairs sat directly through the front doorway, my patient at the top was seated in a small wooden armless chair surrounded by firefighters. An oxygen mask had been place over her nose and mouth helping her breath. Panic was evident on her face as we made eye contact on my way up the stairs. Renato was right behind me with the stair chair. The woman's daughter was a few feet down the hall attempting to reassure her mom that everything would be all right. The crew of Engine 12 knew exactly what needed to be done and wasted no time doing it. I gave what I hoped to be a comforting squeeze to the patients shoulder as I passed, telling her not to worry, we would help her breath and to hang on. The guys were transferring the woman from her chair to ours while I talked to the daughter and got a history.

"She started having a little trouble last night, but it seemed to go away, then she this morning she really started having trouble so we called you. She's really getting worse, is she going to be ok?"

"Has she ever had trouble like this before?" I asked.

"Last year she was in the hospital for two weeks after having a heart attack. The doctor has her on all kinds of medicine."

"What medicine is she on?" I asked.

"They know at the hospital, let's go"

"I need to know, do you have a list?"

"Just get her to the hospital." She said, obviously irritated by my questions. Beyond the woman I saw seven or eight prescription bottles on a dresser in a bedroom.

"Are those hers?"

"For God's sake, yes." She answered, now in a panic. I walked past her and scooped up the bottles. We had carried the patient to the bottom of the stairs and to the back of the rescue where the firefighters were preparing to move her from the stair chair to the stretcher. I entered the rig through the side door and got the truck ready. The first thing I did was turn on the O2. The portable tank that the engine company had her hooked up to was running low. Next, I turned on the EKG machine and got the leads ready. I moved the IV kit to the bench seat as the stretcher was being rolled in. The patient looked worse, now gasping for air. Her lungs were full, immediate treatment imperative. All of the guys on Engine 12 have extensive rescue experience. I passed the EKG leads to Tim who placed them in the right places and asked Renato to start an IV. Trial under fire. One of the other guys had hooked the patient to the pulsox and blood pressure monitor. I had found out from the prescription bottles that her name was Delores. Her pulsox reading was 82% and her BP 240/130. While Renato started the IV, I asked Tim to give her a Nitro tab. Nitroglycerine is used to dilate the arteries and help with blood flow. Tim slipped a 1/150 dose under Delores's tongue, I told her to let it melt, and then put her on a nebulizer treatment. Albuterol was placed in a reservoir, O2 added at approximately 6 Liters/minute, which created a medicated mist that dilates the bronchi. Renato, wiped sweat from his forehead and informed me that the IV was ready. I looked through Delores's medications and found what I was looking for. She took a medication called furosimide, which is a diuretic used to adsorb excess liquid. Her dose was forty-milligrams/ day, our protocols call for us to double the amount during a breathing emergency and administer it through an IV. I drew up eighty mg, pinched the IV line and slowly pushed the drug through, then flushed with normal saline. In a few moments I reassessed her vital signs to see if our ministrations had been effective. In the meantime, the look of relief on Delores's face told me all I needed to know. The stress level decreasing in the back of the truck was like the air being let out of a balloon that was ready to burst. We rechecked her vitals, now 160/100 with a pulse of 100 and a pulsox of 92%. Not great, but a lot better than it was. The most important vital sign was Delores's face. She had relaxed now, relief flooding through her eyes in the form of tears, her breathing returned to normal. Renato looked as though he had just witnessed a miracle. How anybody could think of what we do as ordinary is beyond me, I thought as I wiped the signs of my own relief from my face.

One of the firefighters from Engine 12 drove the rescue over to Our Lady of Fatima, which was the closest hospital from where we were and the Engine followed. Delores's daughter sat on the bench seat and kept an eye on her mom as we made our way to the ER. I observed Renato's reaction as we drove. It was obvious he was reveling in the beautiful feeling you get when you save somebody's life. Delores would have been dead minutes ago if not for our intervention. Renato knew it, yet couldn't believe what he had just done. I think I may have found a replacement for Mike.

I filled out the report while monitoring Delores's vital signs, the facts of what we just accomplished filling the empty paper, but never able to tell the whole story.

PART III

EIGHTEEN

0700 hrs. (7:00 a.m.)

I had ten hours to go. All things considered, it wasn't a bad night. A few hours sleep goes a long way. The light was at the end of the tunnel. Unfortunately, sometimes that light is a train coming at you full speed ahead.

Delores was good hands. Her condition had greatly improved from the time we arrived at her house until she was admitted. I could barely contain Renato's excitement as we drove back to the station. "What a night," he said, still full of adrenaline. "I love Ladder 4, but tonight was unbelievable! We saved that old lady's life! And the kid that got shot! I helped more people tonight than I have since I got hired!"

He had learned a lot and was making a good name for himself department wide but his first night on a rescue was a real eye opener. I hoped he was hooked.

I had to get back to Rescue 1 and relieve Mark, who was in charge of the rescue on B Group. Me and Renato left together. He was tired but still beaming from the night's events.

"Let me know if you ever need a partner," he said, which was music to my ears.

"I just might," I told him, trying not to get too enthusiastic. When the rush wears off after a night like we just had, people sometimes come to their senses and decide they are happier fighting fires, though those fires are becoming few and far between.

We shook hands at the bottom of the stairs, Renato started his Lexus and I cranked up the old Toyota. I was seriously considering leaving the rescue division after Mike left. Training a new partner is hard enough, but it is torture training somebody who would rather be somewhere else. Most of the people who get sent to rescue put their best foot forward and do their best, but their heart is not in it. Renato seemed to truly enjoy the work and wasn't adversely effected by the volume of calls. I kept my fingers crossed. If I left rescue I would lose the overtime and have to get a part time job. The cleaning business was an option but I had hoped to retire my mop. Time would tell. For now I took it day by day and hoped things would work out. Not a foolproof plan but the only one I had.

Traffic was light; I was back in Rescue 1's office ten minutes later.

Mark was lying in the bunk with one eye open, "ready wrapped," a firefighter term for somebody who sleeps with their clothes on.

"How was your night?" he asked. I told him about the shooting. He had already heard most of the story from the people at the ER, but rescue guys like to share the details that nobody else hears.

"This city is nuts," he said, shaking his head as he picked up his things and got ready to head home. His night was busy, "four after," another firefighter term for the number of calls that you have between midnight and shift change.

My energy was holding up, but I had a long way to go. Weekdays are brutally busy. The city's residents are joined by thousands of workers from out of town; the potential for medical emergencies immense. I knew I'd be running all day with little hope for a break. "No time like the present," I said to the empty office, slipping into the bunk, still warm from Mark's body heat. Kind of gross, but at the time I didn't care. Mark gave me the radio and left. I was sound asleep in minutes.

"Rescue 1 and Engine 9 a still alarm."

Here we go.

0915 hrs. (9:15 a.m.)

"Rescue 1 and Engine 9; respond to the Steere House for a possible allergic reaction."

I fumbled for my radio and said,
"Rescue 1 is on the way."
Mike was back in the driver's seat, looking refreshed.
"You look like shit," he said.
"Thank you," I replied. "And fuck you." His laugh filled the small space, infecting me. I was going to miss him.

We left the station, lights activated and siren wailing, quickly making our way as the other vehicles moved to the side of the road. The Steere House is a nursing home located about five miles from the station, right around the corner from Rhode Island Hospital.

I always thought that I wanted to live forever. If I couldn't live forever, I thought one hundred years would do. Now that I have seen how so many of our elderly citizens spend their last few years on earth I have decided that if at all possible I want to die with my boots on. I realize that there are not many alternatives to nursing home care at the end of our years, but I hate to see a person's dignity fade at the end of a long productive life.

My mother lives in a nursing home after suffering a massive stroke in 1996. Her care is the best available, much better than my siblings or I could provide in our homes. Sadly, something is sorely lacking. The elderly once had a position of honor in our society, earned through a life of accomplishment. Now they sit or lay in their beds, heavily medicated revenue producers for nursing home owners. Their days end in a sterile environment full of strangers waiting and hoping in vain for somebody from their past to visit. As time progresses, the staff at the homes become more important than their families. When I can I stop by the nursing home. My job and the odd hours I work afford me the luxury of stopping by whenever it is convenient. Sometimes that is at two in the afternoon, in the middle of visiting hours when everybody is on their toes, other times I'll drop in at two in the morning, surprising the night shift. It keeps people on their toes, though they have never given me a reason to worry about the care my mother receives.

After the stroke she was feisty, even insisted that she be brought home. I thought she had a chance. Instead, her body wore down as time progressed. Her personality slowly disappeared, receding into the shell of her withering body, unable to communicate. Visiting her feels like I've taken my heart out of my chest, squeezed the life out of it like a spent dishrag then threw it onto the floor. I'll sit for a while, she'll look at me with eyes full of intelligence that she can no longer share as I wait for the next call. Sometimes it is quick, and I begin the healing process quickly. Other times an eternity passes before somebody else needs me and my radio breaks the silence in the room. At those times I long for anything to get me out of there. I'll give her hand a squeeze, kiss her on the forehead and walk away. My heart eventually returns to normal, but I think I leave a little on the floor every time I visit. I can only imagine how my mother feels.

The nursing home is filled with characters. I wonder why some of the elderly maintain a lively, optimistic spark while others are filled with resentment. We all lead similar lives; our hearts broken then mended again and again, at times hurting so badly it seems death may be preferable to life. I wonder if the resentful have had their hearts broken too often; their hearts filled with shattered pieces with no room for pain while those more optimistic escape the brunt of heartache most of us bear. Perhaps some are able to deal with grief more efficiently than others, storing the shreds of torn dreams, lost loves and failing health somewhere where they stay forever buried.

I placed the blue canvas med bag onto the stretcher and Mike and I worked our way through the front doors of the facility and into the lobby. Inside the blue canvas bag is everything needed for handling an on scene emergency. An IV set-up, all of the drugs we are licensed to carry, intubation equipment, a bag/valve device and trauma dressings are inside.

A grand piano, beautiful floral arrangements, sofas and chairs fill the lobby. A big, yellow alley cat slept on the grand piano. I rubbed the top of his head on my way past him; he was asleep and barely stirred.

"Engine 9 to Fire Alarm, advise rescue we have a twenty-five year old female, possible allergic reaction."

"Rescue 1 received," I said into the mike. I thought I heard Pat, the officer of Engine 9 say a twenty-five year old but was sure he was mistaken. Ninety-five is the age of most of our patients here.

They were on the second floor so we headed to the elevator, pushed the right buttons and began our ascent. The door opened to three firefighters hovering over a person lying on her back in the hallway, covered with a sheet. I was impressed with our guys' dedication and efficiency. They did everything possible making the patient more comfortable. They monitored vital signs, gave supplemental oxygen and treated her with the utmost kindness and care. I couldn't recall seeing this much enthusiasm for a patient since the last time we went to the Foxy Lady to treat a dancer who had fainted. The closer to the patient I got, the clearer the situation became. She was indeed twenty-five, beautiful, and covered with hives, but breathing normally. She was embarrassed by all of the attention.

"What happened?" I asked her after fighting my way through the firefighters.

"I took some new medication this morning, an antibiotic," she explained. "When I got to work I began to itch all over. Then I noticed these hives."

Red bumps and welts appeared on her face and arms, probably under her clothes as well. I hoped there were no hives internally. She looked as though she spent the night in a jungle without a mosquito net. I scratched an imaginary itch on my arm.

"Are you having trouble breathing?" I asked.

"No, but I am really itchy."

"We're going to take you to the hospital so they can check you out," I told her while scratching my head.

"Do I have to go? I think I'll be fine in a little while."

"I think you might start to have trouble breathing. If your airway swells up, you could be in a lot of trouble." She recognized the situation as potentially serious and acquiesced.

"All right, let's go," she agreed reluctantly.

She tried talking us into letting her walk, but we insisted on putting her on the stretcher. The elderly residents got a kick out of seeing one of their caregivers on their end of things, even if only for a little while. I'm only too happy to give them a little entertainment.

The guys from Engine 9 helped us get the patient, Sarah into the truck.

"Thanks for the help guys, we'll take it from here," I said.

"Anytime," Pat replied.

"Take care, Sarah," said Ben, grinning from ear to ear. If you ever need anything, you know who to call."

"You guys have been great," said Sarah as I closed the rear doors of the rescue.

The firefighters reluctantly went back to the engine, their job well done. Mike and I had some work to do before transporting.

"Quit scratching yourself," said Mike. "It's only a subliminal suggestion."

"I'm not scratching," I replied, taking the tip of my finger out of the ear I was scratching. If somebody started to yawn I'd be in big trouble.

"We're going to give you some oxygen and an IV just to be safe," I told Sarah.

"Is all of this necessary?"

"Why are nurses always the worst patients?" I asked her.

With a knowing conspiratorial look she replied, "No worse than firemen."

Mike hooked her up to the oxygen and started the IV while I drew fifty milligrams of dipenhydremine from a vial into a syringe. Dipenhydremene, better known as Benadryl is one of the drugs we use to treat allergic reactions. With the IV set, her vitals signs checked and oxygen being delivered through a nasal cannula, Sarah was ready to go. I pushed the Benadryl through the IV line and we were on our way. The drug worked fast. Sarah felt the itching subside before we arrived at Rhode Island Hospital. So did I.

The mid-morning rush was on at the ER. Seven rescues were parked in the cramped space yet Mike managed to squeeze into the spot closest to the door. He shut down the engine, got out of the drivers seat and opened the rear door letting the bright sunshine filter in. Sarah was much better, the Benadryl helped. She tried again to escape the clutches of the ER by claiming that she was fine. I almost relented, but in the end wheeled her through the ER doors so they could start the process of her care. There wasn't much that the ER staff could do now that the Benadryl has been administered and was effective. She would have to wait for a few hours while they kept an eye on her airway. Sometimes when the drug wears off, the symptoms return. Airways close incredibly fast during an allergic reaction. I've seen patients breathing one minute, their airway completely blocked the next. It is a tragedy that happens all too often, often to the young and healthy.

A police officer working a detail at a local festival was stung by a bee one beautiful day last summer. He wasn't aware of his bee sting allergy because he had never been stung. He ignored his symptoms as his heart rate increased, his hands began to swell and hives appeared. His airway closed quickly, he fell to the ground gasping for a breath of the same air the festival goers surrounding him breathed with ease. He was thirty-seven years old and left a wife and a couple of kids. This was the best place for Sarah until the situation cleared up.

The patients were stacking up, almost out the door. I saw a few regulars; Darryl, wearing his old clothes and a stupid grin was being escorted off of the property by security. He would be back by noon, depending on how quickly he sold his stolen papers.

Rescue 5 backed into the bay before we left, taking one of the spots just vacated. Rescues come and go all day. When their truck stopped I opened the rear doors to say hello. Theresa was in back with another regular, this one a creepy homeless guy that claims to have chest pains a few times a week. He enjoys getting stuck with needles. He knows all of the women on rescue by name, which I find disturbing. Theresa can't help being nice to everybody that she comes in contact with, I hate seeing people like this guy take advantage of that kindness. She is more than capable of handling herself, and this was her patient, so I let it rest.

I sometimes think it is my responsibility to look out for the new people on the other rescues. Most of the senior, experienced rescue officers are burned out by the sheer volume of calls and have left the division to join the fire fighting force. Junior people, fresh out of the training academy have been forced to fill the vacancies, most with a lot of EMT training but very little street experience. Some of them have only six months on the job. Rookies in Providence are in charge of some of the busiest rescues in the country. These "kids" have proven themselves time and time again. They have been exposed to horrors most people will never experience, have performed admirably, in some cases heroically and continue to do the job better than anybody has the right to expect.

"Hey, Theresa, how are you?" I asked while helping her move the "patient", a three hundred-pound hypochondriac out of the truck. I'm always happy to see Theresa. Her charm and attitude is contagious.

"Dude, what's up?" she responded, her smile lighting up the back of the dingy rescue. She looks and sounds more like a California surfer girl than a firefighter in Providence.

"I think we're getting breakfast. I'm sure Mike is due for his hourly feeding," I said.

"Where are you going, we'll meet you," she said while we wheeled the patient from the rescues rear doors.

"Brook Street for some Mexican Bagels," I said. There is a bagel shop across the street from the Brook Street fire station run by Mexican people that make the best bagels in the city. They also make breakfast burritos and nachos, but their bagels are what make me come back.

"We'll meet you there!" she said. Her partner, Tim eats as much as Mike. The three of them never gain a pound. There is a calendar in Rhode Island featuring "buff" firefighters. Both Tim and Mike have graced the pages. I could too if I wanted, if I wasn't old, fat and ugly.

Tim and Theresa brought their patient into the ER and Mike and I went to the bagel store. I put us at the mercy of the dispatchers when I keyed the mike and went in service. The chances of us actually meeting Tim and Theresa for breakfast was slim, but we try to make the job a little more enjoyable.

NINETEEN

"Where are you going?" I asked Mike as he turned the truck away from the Brook Street Bagel Store.

"Dunkin Donuts," he replied matter of factly.

"We're going to Brook Street," I said, asserting my rank.

"You always get two bagels when we go there," Mike replied, not impressed.

"I want two bagels."

"If you quit complaining about how fat you're getting we would go to Brook Street."

"If you mind your own business I won't fire you!"

"Fire away," he says while laughing hysterically. "I need the time off." I have to laugh along.

Mike stopped in front of the Dunkin Donut shop and said, "What do you want, I'm buying."

"You bought yesterday, I've got it. The usual?" I asked.

"No, just a coffee, Art made pancakes while you were sleeping."

"Why didn't you wake me up?"

"You would have killed me."

"Now I'm really going to kill you!" I love pancakes.

I crossed Eddy Street and waited in line. I only got one bagel and Mike his coffee. We had a lot to do today between runs. The truck needed fuel, and a trip to the repair shop to fix a thing that holds the stretcher in place were a few things on the list. Rescue 1 was less than a year old but already signs of wear and tear showed. We also had to go to a medical oxygen supply depot. The truck is equipped with a large O2 tank that lasts a couple of weeks and some smaller portable tanks, all were almost empty.

"What time does Venda open?" I asked Mike while handing him his drink.

"They're open now do you want to head over there?"

"Nah, let's go back to quarters and get the maintenance out of the way, we'll go this afternoon," I said.

"You're going to forget."

"Never happen."

Mike asks, "Why do you eat manicotti on Easter anyway. What's wrong with ham?"

"It's an Italian thing," I explained. "There'll be plenty of ham and all of that, but Cheryl and the girls like pasta so we always get something to go with the gravy."

"Giving the girls what the want. Smart man," Mike said as we headed toward the station.

Fire stations and the apparatus they hold don't take care of themselves. Back at the barn spring-cleaning was under way. Captain Healy was a true taskmaster at this time of year. He learned how to clean a fire station from the volunteer firefighters in his hometown, Warren, RI and hasn't changed a thing. Hot water, soap and elbow grease are all that mattered to him during spring cleaning. He had posted a cleaning list on the bulletin board a few weeks ago, the work expected to be done in an expedient manner. Each group was responsible for a section of the station. The Captain of the House designates the assignments. Having the Captain on our shift should have been a good thing, but Captain Healy marches to the beat of his own drummer. He decided to give us most of the work, "to be fair."

Rescue 1 was responsible for the apparatus floor bathroom and two of the offices in the living quarters. Mike took care of the bathroom while I started to do the offices. Whether or not we finished our tasks was up to the rescue gods. When we need them to chime in, they never do. I filled a bucket with hot soapy water and began to clean.

Downstairs, I heard all hell break loose. Shouts and hysterical laughter were coming through the holes in the floor where the sliding poles are. Being a cagey old veteran, I knew this could only mean one thing: WATER FIGHT! No respectable spring cleaning would be complete without one.

Mike was outnumbered. I knew that the guys from Engine 13 were ganging up on him. Nothing is fair when it comes to water fights. The only rule is, "THERE ARE NO RULES!" Too bad for Engine 13, they have forgotten that I am upstairs, and have years of water fight experience. I filled three big pans with water and placed them on a windowsill in the dorm, directly over Engine 13's overhead door. I left the weapons on the ledge and retreated to my locker.

Inside was a package of water balloons left over from last year. I filled four of them from the sink in the kitchen. Once through, I booby-trapped the kitchen sprayer by holding it open with a rubber band wrapped around the handle. In the bathroom, I pointed the showerheads directly in the path of whoever turned the lever. I strategically placed the balloons on the top landing of the stairs. I was ready to join the battle.

I was the only one on the upper level and used that to my advantage. The guys from Engine 13 were on the ramp, buckets of water or hoses in hand, waiting to ambush Mike. Captain Healy, a cagey veteran himself was nowhere to be seen, but I couldn't worry about him just then. If I could quietly open the window above them I'd have a clean shot. If they heard me I'd be good as good as dead. I could only see two of them, which left the other two unaccounted for. Not good. The potential for surround and drown tactics from the enemy was growing as each valuable second ticked. This was a battle that I hadn't anticipated. Without proper communication with Mike, success of the entire operation was in jeopardy. We had never been to war together, but I hoped his instincts would see us through. I gently pushed the window up. It hadn't been opened since the fall and got stuck. I felt my heart pounding out of my chest and hoped the enemy couldn't hear it thumping. Sweat poured down my forehead and into my eyes, blinding me. The window finally gave, but not without a loud "crack!" I jumped from my position, and as the targets looked up, I unloaded with everything I had.

Direct Hit!

My first mission accomplished, I ran to the top of the stairs to head off the counterattack. If my calculations were correct, Mike would flank them from behind, brandishing the hose we use to wash the trucks. I should make it to the landing in time to retrieve the water grenades and we'd have them in crossfire. I left my position and headed for the stairs.

"Engine 13 and Rescue 1 a still Alarm."

1158 hrs. (11:58 a.m.)

War is hell. My brilliant plan had to wait. I aborted the mission and headed for the 0915 truck. An uneasy truce had been declared.

Rescue 1 and Engine 13, head over to 359 Montgomery Ave for an elderly woman with a possible broken leg.

"Rescue 1 on the way."

We followed the engine, leaving the battlefield and headed toward the incident. Another hi-rise, this one was located close to the city of Cranston in a residential area. The engine flew toward the destination, its federal siren wailing and air horn disturbing the noontime serenity of South Providence. We followed behind at a safe distance, not making nearly as much racket. When traveling through intersections the little white truck behind the big red one is often not seen and collisions happen.

The engine pulled past the front door of the building, us right behind them. A few people mingled around the lobby. Mike and I wheeled the stretcher past the crowd.

"All right ladies, who's coming with us?" he asked the members of the housecoat brigade. They chuckled and said, "not us today."

"Seven B," said one of the ladies.

"She probably tripped over her beer can," said another, much to the delight of the crowd.

"Be nice," I told them as the elevator door closed.

There were six firefighters crammed into the elevator, five of them soaked. The elevator stopped on the seventh floor and we filed out, our war temporarily forgotten. The door to 7B was open; we left the stretcher in the hall and filed in. Sitting on the arm of an old gray couch was a woman in her late sixties. She rubbed the bottom of her leg. I let Captain Healy do the talking because he does whether I let him or not.

"What's the problem?" he asked, all business.

"I tripped and broke my fucking leg," she responded.

"How do you know it's broken?" asked the Captain.

"Because it fucking hurts," she responded.

I got the stretcher from the hall and wheeled it to our patient. She didn't waste a second, hopped right on. Her apartment was full of smoke and there was a lit cigarette in an ashtray on the edge of a wood coffee table that was covered with burn marks. Empty beer cans littered the cheap cigarette burned carpet, a wastebasket was spilling over with empties.

"What is your name?" I asked.

"Gertrude," she replied.

"Let's get you to the hospital so they can get a look at your leg."

"No shit," she said, folding her arms across her chest waiting for us to put out her cigarettes and lock the door. The guys from Engine 13 secured her place while Mike and I transported.

My cell phone rang on the way to the hospital. I knew it was Cheryl, but hoped Gertrude did not.

"Rescue 1, go ahead with your message," I answered in an official tone.

"Why do you answer the phone with a patient in the truck?" she asked.

"We've got a sixty year old female, possible multiple fractures to her lower legs, we'll need a trauma room," I said.

"You are an idiot. Call me later."

"Roger that, over and out."

I put the phone back in my top pocket and evaluated my patient. Her lower left leg had a small bruise, nothing more.

"I don't think you broke it, Gertrude, it may be just a bruise," I said.

"How the fuck do you know that?" she asked.

"Because I am an EMT," I responded.

"Big fucking deal."

"Why do you swear so much?" I asked her.

"Why the fuck do you care?"

"I don't, I was just making conversation."

"Does it bother you?" she asked. I think she actually cared if it did.

"Not really."

"Honestly, I don't realize that I'm swearing," she explained. I don't think anybody has listened to her for some time. "My husband died six months ago and I have been talking to myself since. I don't notice and those assholes at the hi-rise never talk to me so fuck them."

"Have you lived there for long?"

"We moved in about a year ago, then Harv died. He died in his sleep, nice and peaceful. We used to live in a big house on Alabama Ave, big yard, nice house you know. We never should have sold it, I think that's what killed him. Our neighbors had eleven kids, used to drive us crazy. It's funny; you don't miss nothing till it's gone. Those kid's weren't all that bad. Some of em anyway."

As we approached Rhode Island hospital, Gertrude appeared lost in her memories. It appears that she has endured her share of heartache. I hoped there was still room for joy between the cracks. Maybe someday happiness will find her again. She didn't swear once while she told me her story. I wondered if she realized it.

TWENTY

Annie was at the triage when we brought Gertrude in for treatment. Annie and I shared a love of Bruce Springsteen. Springsteen fans usually have a lot of soul and compassion so I knew Gertrude was in good hands.

The stretcher wobbled a little when Mike put it into the back of the rescue because the thing that holds it in place was loose. We needed to get to the repair shop soon or it would fall right off.

"Are they making lunch?" I asked Mike.

"Chicken Caesar," he said.

"Think they'll have olives in it this time?"

"I hope so."

"When are you going to Engine 15," I asked.

"Not this week but the week after," he said. "I feel pretty bad leaving, we've had a lot of fun."

"Believe me, I'm going to miss you. I think you're doing the right thing though. Everybody on this job needs to see some fire up close or you may as well work for a private ambulance company. You'll do great over there, the officer is a good guy, and when your bid is up you're always welcome back here."

"That's what I'm hoping. A couple of years on a fire truck and I'll be eligible to take the fire lieutenants test. Then I'll come back to rescue. These nitwits would miss me too much if I'm gone too long," he said.

We were almost back to the station when Engine 13 was called to Oxford Street for a man unconscious on the sidewalk. No Providence rescues were in service, the 13's would have to wait up to a half an hour for a rescue from a surrounding town to respond and transport. Being conscientious guys, we jumped right in.

"We better get that or the 13's won't have time to make lunch," I said to Mike.

"Let's go," he said and turned the truck around.

1345 hrs. (12:45 p.m.)

"Rescue 1 to fire alarm, clearing Rhode Island, we'll handle Oxford.

"Received, Rescue 1, we received this call from a cell phone caller."

"Roger, on the way."

I put the mike back in its cradle and leaned back in my seat. The long hours were starting to take their toll. I had less than five hours to go yet it seemed like an eternity.

There are still some kind souls that will stop and help a person in need. The rest call 911 from cell phones and let somebody else do the work. It's neater that way and there is no guilt; a person needed help and help was on the way.

It only took a minute to reach our victim. He sat in a gravel pit next to the road in a construction site, under a bridge leaning against the abutment. Mike wheeled the truck beside him, I got out and closed the door, the trucks above us on Route 95 shook the ground, and the sound of the door slamming shut woke him. His bloodshot eyes popped open at the sound, he jumped to his feet and slowly walked away from me. I easily caught up and stopped him.

"Are you alright?" I asked.

"I'm fine, why don't you leave me alone?" he responded miserably.

"A concerned citizen drove past you and thought you needed assistance. They called 911 from their cell phone," I explained.

"Why don't they mind their business?" he asked me.

"I don't know. Are you all right?"

"If people left me alone I would be."

"Have a nice day then." I walked back to the truck. I wondered what happened to this guy to make him wander around the city in the middle of the day. He didn't appear homeless, if he was he hadn't been for long. He was another lost soul in a city full of them. How could such loneliness exist with so many people living so close to each other? Maybe he and Gertrude will meet. I thought they would be good for each other.

"What's up with that guy?" asked Mike.

"I don't know. I hope he doesn't turn into a regular."

"None of the regulars have died lately, there's no room."

"I heard they're taking applications in case there's a vacancy," I said sarcastically.

Our callous comments made me think back to a few years ago. I was new to the rescue division. A homeless man's plight caught my attention and I wrote about him. The local paper published the story in the Sunday paper as a human interest story. Few people were interested.

I didn't think I cared. The frequency of the calls made it hard to care. Nuisance calls made up a large part of our routine. Spaced between medical emergencies, calls from the city's underground emerged. Sivine Thatch made a lot of calls. He was a nuisance. One of many.

The tone from the stations PA system was the new alternative to the traditional fire bell. Rather than being shocked into action by a loud bell like our predecessors, we were alerted to an emergency by a soothing tone. This sound woke you from a deep sleep as well as any bell. During a thirty-eight hour shift, the peaceful tone becomes your worst enemy. The stations quiet is shattered by the "relaxing" noise as your body vibrates from its sound. It sounds hourly, twenty-four hours a day.

"Rescue One, respond to 1288 Broad Street for an intoxicated male," boomed the voice from the loudspeaker. *That voice alerted us to tragedies other people's lives far too often. Annoyed that I had to respond to another "nuisance" call, I was relieved that a real tragedy was not what waited at 1288 Broad Street.*

I knew from experience that Sivine would be waiting, full of cheap vodka, spewing venom from his filthy mouth. He was a small man, five feet tall, usually dressed in old doctor's scrubs. Periodically the staff at the area hospitals cleaned and dressed him in whatever cast off clothing they could find, usually donations or forgotten items from previous patients. Not long ago, I had transported him to RI Hospital's detox unit. When his blood alcohol level became acceptable, he was released back into the city's waiting arms. The hospital staff knew he wouldn't be gone for long. They were aware of Sivine and others like him.

There are countless homeless alcoholics in the city. When they receive their disability checks from the government, they quickly change the cash into alcohol. After consuming as much as their tired bodies will allow, some find a pay phone and call 911 requesting medical assistance, others they collapse where they stood and a concerned citizen will make the call for them. Either way, one of the city's five rescue units gets called to haul them off the street and out of the tax paying publics eye. We would load them into our trucks, which we cleaned and sanitized diligently after each run, and take them in. Most of the time they left us with vomit, urine and feces or a combination of the three on the floor and stretcher as a reminder of their visit with us. The smell lingered for hours. It saddened the rescue crews and striped them of their morale seeing their hard work and professionalism being wasted time and time again on the same patients and their self inflicted sickness.

After transferring care of the patients to the emergency room, they would be put into hospital beds, cleaned and fed, then put into the detox room until they were ready to leave. The taxpayer got the bill. Most of the alcoholics know how the system works, and the ones that don't quickly learned how easily the system could be abused. They would make promises of sobriety with a grin on their faces as they left the hospital. Nobody believed them.

The path to Sivine from the station is a road that I traveled often. Triple deckers loom on either side of the street. Litter fills the gutters which the rats call home. I turned down one of the streets that cut through the South Providence neighborhood between Broad and Allen's Avenue. Like most of the inner city, this street is worn from years of neglect. Some homes showed the pride of the people inside. Sadly, most did not. When I allowed it, I recalled the horrors I had witnessed on these streets. Over the years I have seen a lifetime of bloodshed and heartache. Today, I have a job to do. Sivine waited.

I pulled the rescue next to the curb where he sat on the filthy sidewalk. This time his pants were around his knees. I approached him, he spit at me and screamed, "You go away!" I put on some latex gloves, and with the help of my partner carried him to the back of the rescue.

"I don't care for you!" He shouted in broken English as we placed him on the floor of the truck. On the way to detox he rambled of his hatred of America. He wanted to go back to Vietnam. I did not think that he would be alive long enough to make the trip.

I met Sivine in 1996. Alcohol and despair were the only constant factors in his life. I didn't know why he lived in Providence. I did know that he would never leave. His lifestyle had destroyed his ability to make rational decisions. He could no longer take care of himself. He spent his days roaming Broad Street, one notorious for violence. Nobody bothered him; they knew that he had nothing to offer. The few nights he didn't spend in the hospital he slept in a burned out garage located behind some *trees, a few yards from the street. People had tried to help him but he pushed them away. Eventually, nobody bothered, he had become a waste of time and effort.*

At the hospital, I brought the rescue to the emergency room door, parked it and wheeled a bed from inside to the rear of the truck. I opened the door, the smell of unwashed humanity filtered into the night. Feces and urine covered Sivine's legs. As we wheeled our human cargo past the ER staff we were met with a mixture of laughter, sadness and revulsion. Again I heard the chorus, "Welcome back Sivine." He spat onto the floor. "I don't care for you!" he shouted at anybody who got near him. The routine of caring for him got underway.

While leaving the triage area where Sivine had been placed, I covered him with a blanket. Looking up at me with empty helpless eyes he simply said, in English, "thank you."

As night progressed toward dawn and the end of my shift, the look of empty despair in Sivine's eyes came back to haunt me. I remembered joking with my partner about being better off when Sivine died. One January, we found him in a snow bank, unconscious and frostbitten. I don't know how he survived. The temperature outside was in the low teens. He should have died that day just as surely as the day he was found passed out in a field on an oppressively hot July day, his body temperature an astonishing 106 degrees. We started a pool to guess when we would be rid of him.

We brought our final patient of the night, a 64 year old woman suffering from a seizure into the ER. I was shocked at what I saw. A clean, smiling Sivine sat on his hospital bed. A small crowd of workers and patients stood around as he entertained them, animatedly telling stories. Later, I discovered he spoke fluent French, Spanish and Vietnamese as well as broken English. His audience thought he was quite charming. He looked me in the eye. I looked away.

I thought of Sivine during my days off. I wondered if the spark of life that he showed in the hospital could be a new beginning for him. I honestly hoped that it would.

It was business as usual when I returned to work. By mid morning we had responded to four or five emergencies and another homeless alcoholic. Somehow, I managed to take a seat in the hospital's break room. The conversation there ranged from the hockey game the previous night to a bad date over the weekend and everything in between. One subject got only a small mention. Sivine lay dying.

A call from a concerned citizen came in requesting help for an unconscious person lying in the street. The rescue crew working that day found Sivine. Whatever spark of life there once was now was extinguished. The crew did what they are paid to do, they brought him back to life with CPR and other advanced life support techniques. They managed to get his heart beating, but his brain had died a long time ago. He lay in a coma for a few days before the plug was pulled. I thought of going to his room to see him but never did. Sivine died alone in his hospital room. At least he did not die on the street.

I searched the obituaries for a while to find some more about him, but no obituary was ever printed. Nobody cared. Sivine was gone. At times while dealing with "nuisance calls," I think of Sivine and the spark of life that he showed on the last day that I saw him. His memory has helped me to find some compassion that I hope I'm not losing.

There are still plenty of homeless alcoholics rummaging around the city. Some manage to sober up; most die broken and alone. As annoying as they are, I know and genuinely like some of them. Their familiarity is welcome. It helps knowing what to expect in a job full of the unexpected.

TWENTY-ONE

"Rescue 1 a special signal."

1252 hrs. (12:52 p.m.)

"Rescue 1, respond to Broad at Dudley, Engine 10 on scene at a street box with an intoxicated male."

"Rescue 1 on the way."

Mike activated the lights and siren and we were off. Street boxes are a throwback to the days before cell phones. To alert the fire department of a fire while away from a phone, the street box was used. Every few blocks there is a red box wired to the fire alarm office waiting to be of use. False alarms emanating from these boxes are abundant. Slowly the boxes are being removed until someday they will be gone. Even now they are coveted collectors items.

I saw Engine 10 in the distance as we turned onto Broad Street from Oxford. The crew was standing outside of their truck talking to three men. We pulled our vehicle beside them.

"What's going on?" I asked Dan, standing a few feet from the crowd.

"This asshole pulled the box because his legs hurt," he responded while pointing his thumb over his shoulder in the general direction of the people standing around the street box. "We should arrest him for pulling a false alarm."

The guilty party was sitting on a cement retaining wall a few feet from the alarm box, obviously intoxicated. His friends came over to me to plead their case

"His legs hurt real bad, he ain't walking," said one man, horrifically skinny, his scraggly gray beard full of crumbs.

"You got to take him to the hospital," said another fellow, this one in a motorized wheelchair and wearing beautiful snakeskin boots with red flames stitched on the sides.

"Where did you get those boots?" I asked him.

"Don't you be worryin bout my boots. My boy can't walk, you best be worryin bout him."

"If he can't walk, how did he get here?" I asked.

"He's here that's all you need to know, now git him in the truck and take him to the hospital."

"The hospital is only half a mile away, why didn't you call a cab or take a bus if you're so concerned."

"Cause you are free, he don't got no money to be takin a bus."

"He has money for booze and cigarettes."

"Are you gonna take him or not?"

"How bout I take you instead?" I asked greybeard.

"What you talkin' bout?"

"You're intoxicated, maybe you should go to detox. Or better yet, maybe I'll call the police and have you arrested for pulling a false alarm."

"Fuck you man." He walked away, the fight taken out of him.

"What you wanna fuck with us poor folk for?" flaming boots asked me. "We didn't do nothin, just tryin to help a friend in need."

"Why don't you help yourself."

I was getting tired. Normally I would just bring the drunken man to the hospital without any fuss. Today the abuse really bothered me. My patience had worn out and I was taking it out on these people. They were wrong, but I was wasting my time arguing with them and I knew it. Engine 10 had already left the scene and Mike was putting the drunk into the truck. He had witnessed my mood swings before and only intervened when I got irrational. For now he let me waste my time trying to talk sense into the senseless.

I got in the truck with Mike and the patient. He was sitting on the bench seat, Mike was taking his vital signs.

"What's your name?" I asked, beginning the procedure.

"Ivan." He responded.

"Date of birth?"

"Ten, five fifty four," he said automatically.

"Do you have any medical problems?"

"Yeah. I was in an accident ten years ago and hurt my back. I'm waiting for a settlement."

"What's wrong with your legs?"

"They hurt."

"How long have they hurt for?"

"Ten years."

"Are you taking any medication?"

"Yeah, Vicodin but I ran out."

Bingo. The "patient" wanted painkillers. He has probably been living on them for years. "Beans" as Vicodin is sometimes called on the street produces euphoria in the person taking the drug whether he is in pain or not. They sell on the street for five dollars each.

"Do you have any allergies to medicine?"

"Yeah, Tylenol and Advil" He said. If he was allergic to Tylenol and Advil I'll eat the rescue. He was narrowing the options for the doctor to prescribe, knowing how the game is played.

Mike had moved to the front of the truck and headed for Rhode Island Hospital. Ivan will get his painkillers, I'm sure. Vicodin is extremely addictive, some people will do anything to get some.

The hospital was less than a mile away so we were there in no time. Every stretcher was full, the wait five to six hours for routine care, immediate for emergencies. Terry was waiting at the desk. I gave her my report, she listened to me then interviewed the patient. I was impressed by her professionalism. I have become cynical after only a few years on rescue, Terry just celebrated her twenty-fifth anniversary in the ER and treats every patient who comes her way the with the same care and respect I imagine she did on her first day. Being surrounded by good people helps me keep things in perspective. She didn't know it, but her example stayed with me for the rest of the day, making me better at what I do.

TWENTY-TWO

At the station we sat around the table eating chicken Caesar salad. Nothing ever tasted so good. The water fight was forgotten, food was all that mattered. The TV in the corner was tuned to the Senate hearings regarding intelligence failures and the War in Iraq. Condelisa Rice was on the hot seat but I was too tired and hungry to pay attention.

"Why didn't you cut the lettuce smaller?" Steve asked Arthur, today's cook.

"Any bigger and you could have put the whole head in the bowl," added Jay.

"If you used the bowl Mike's wife puts over his head when she cuts his hair you could have fit in a whole field of lettuce," contributed Captain Healy.

"The reason I left the lettuce in large pieces is so the dressing could properly adhere to the leaves," said Arthur who immediately returned to eating his salad.

"All I know is lettuce gives me gas," said Mike as he let one rip, drawing groans from everybody in the room. Mike was in his glory, bathing in the pungent aroma surrounding him while he continued to eat.

"This is the ultimate compliment to the chef," he said and let another one go.

"What is the matter with you?" I asked him, moving to the other table on the other side of the room.

I had three hours to go. A good lunch helped my spirits considerably. After eating everybody pitched in and cleaned the dishes. I could have used a shower but doubted if the rescue gods would permit one. There is no worse feeling that getting into a nice hot shower, soaping up and then hearing the tone go off.

Before I put my plate into the dishwasher I brought it to the sink to rinse. I turned the faucet on and was rewarded with a spray of water directly in my face. I couldn't believe I had fallen victim to my own friendly fire. The guys thought this was the funniest thing they had ever seen. So did I. I retreated to my office, wiped my face, took my cell phone out of my top pocket and closed the door. I had gotten my shower.

"Hey, babe, how's things?"

"Great, I miss you."

"Me too, I'll be home soon."

"Are you tired?"

"Nah, I feel great."

"I'll bet."

"I've only got a few more hours to go."

"I'm sorry you have to work so much," Cheryl said.

"You've got nothing to be sorry about." I meant it.

When I met Cheryl, I was bartending at a local restaurant. She got a job there as a waitress. It was only a matter of time that we were together. Two people couldn't have hit it off better. Within a few months we were dating, a year later I moved in with her and her two girls. Eventually we married. We raised the girls together, they are my daughters. They call me Michael. Years ago, Brittany, the younger of the two was asked why she didn't call me dad; she thought for a second, tilted her head and said, "Because Dad and

Michael mean the same thing." Any doubt of their love for me disappeared that day.

In addition to working at the restaurant, Cheryl worked a few days a week cleaning houses. I started to go along with her. One thing led to another, before we knew it we had a successful cleaning business going. At one point we had twenty-eight accounts. We bought a tiny house, worked together and were well on our way. We never hired anybody to do the work, we did it ourselves. The money was good but the work demanding. Cleaning houses five days a week, then doing a few offices on the weekends eventually takes its toll. We were both pulling in shifts at the restaurant a few nights a week as well. We knew we couldn't take the pace forever, but kept plugging along.

I had been applying for employment with fire departments of local cities for years, never expecting to get hired but always hoping. After years of hard work and perseverance, I was accepted into the Providence Fire Department's forty-second training academy. Cheryl enrolled in court reporting school. She did well and worked incredibly hard for three long years. She sat in a corner of our little house for hours every day working on her speed. Two nights a week she packed up her briefcase and court-reporting machine and drove to Cranston for class. The curriculum was grueling. Ninety percent of those who start the program will never finish. Saturdays she went to the community college to take related courses. She aced the Medical Terminology, Law and English courses and kept pace with or surpassed her classmates.

In her fourth year she started to have difficulty concentrating. Then her fingers went numb. It became more and more difficult for her to keep her speed without making mistakes. One night at dinner she calmly informed us that she had been diagnosed with Multiple Sclerosis. The disease ended her court-reporting dream. We kept the cleaning business but cut way back. MS is a cruel disease. It takes the vitality out of the best years of your life, and then punches your loved ones in the face.

We lost most of Cheryl's paycheck. Part of the reason I am on Rescue is the overtime. The lack of people on the department willing to do the work creates more opportunity to work extra shifts. We still have a few cleaning accounts and do a better job than any "professional" company out there. Cheryl is the heart and soul of the operation and works herself to exhaustion making sure the jobs are done right. Her courage is remarkable and keeps me going when I feel sorry for myself after a long shift. As tired as I get, it pales in comparison to the ravages of living with Multiple Sclerosis.

"I'll see you when you get home," she says.

"Soon."

"Love you, bye." She hung up before I could say anything.

I hit the couch and fall asleep instantly.

"Attention Engine 10, Engine 8, Engine 13, Ladder 5, Ladder 2, Special Hazards, Battalion 2 and Rescue 1, a still box."

Before the speaker stopped vibrating, we were in the trucks waiting for the second round. Sometimes you just know when it's for real.

"Attention Engine's 10, 8 and 13, Ladders 5 and 2, Special Hazards, Battalion 2 and Rescue 1, respond to 184 Hamilton Street for a report of an occupied house fire."

We roared out of the station, following Engine 13. Every truck dispatched to a still box has a job to do, every firefighter on the way to the scene, rookies and veterans alike go over in their heads what waits. The only definite is that the unexpected will occur, but our training and experience overcome that. Plan "B" we call it. Our first job is to follow procedures that have been in place for decades. Every fire crew has a job; everybody's safety depends on each crew doing theirs with no delay or screw-up. When there are screwups, we fix them fast.

Engine 10 arrived on scene and gave the initial report.

"Engine 10 to fire alarm, heavy smoke condition."

Firefighters donned their Scott airpacks, checked their pass devices, purge valves and Kevlar straps. From all directions fire apparatus converged on the scene. What looked to an outsider like madness was actually controlled chaos to the experienced firefighters.

"Engine 10 to fire alarm, Code Red!"

Definite house fire. We flew through the streets of Providence praying nobody was home. At this time of day a lot of kids were home from school, parents at work and no supervision.

Engine 10 pulled their truck past the burning structure, leaving room for Ladder 5 to set up their aerial ladder. Keith and Roland from the 10's took a line from the back of their truck and made their way toward the house, Weathers stayed at the pump panel to provide water. Dan, the officer surveyed the scene doing a size-up until a chief officer arrived so he could join his men as they entered the burning building.

"Engine 10 to fire alarm, three story wood frame, possibly occupied. Fire on the third floor, side 1."

"Message received, Battalion 2 on scene, establishing Hamilton command."

Battalion 2 took control of the fireground. All communications went through him.

While Engine 10 stretched their initial attack line through the rear door and up the stairs toward the fire on the third floor, Ladder 5 set up in front of the house and raised their aerial ladder to the peak. Their goal was to "get the roof'" meaning to get a hole in the highest point to ventilate.

"Engine 8 to command. We have a hydrant; will take care of the water supply."

"Engine 10, charge my line!" Dan's voice was distorted by the mask on the airpack he wore, but understandable. He and his crew were in the thick of things

"Message received," said the chief. Engines 10 and 8 went to work. Two men from the 8's dressed the hydrant, putting ports on the outlets enabling four three inch feeder lines to be connected if necessary. Another firefighter took two three inch feeders from the back of the engine and gave the command to go to Engine 8's driver to move. The hydrant was properly dressed, two feeders hooked up, two ports ready to go if needed and the feeder lines on the way to Engine 10's pump. The driver of Engine 8 helped Engine 10's pump operator hook up the feeders to the intake valves on the pump panel, and then radioed the chief.

"Turn in the feeders."

The men at the hydrant turned the spindle of the hydrant thirteen or fourteen revolutions, opening the gate all the way. The feeders filled with water, expanding and slithering down the street toward Engine 10's pump.

Engine 10 had found the fire. After dragging two-hundred feet of inch and ¾ line up three flights of narrow winding stairs, they fought their way into the third floor apartment. Dan forced the heavily bolted door with his halligan tool. Through the thick blinding smoke and toward the rear of the apartment they went, sensing the heat, experience guiding their moves. They had to crouch lower and lower, the exposed skin on Dan's ears burned, but didn't blister, providing a primitive temperature gauge. He would feel if flashover was imminent and back his guys out. His ears would have to be burning for him to give the order to evacuate. Conditions inside the burning house improved slightly letting the guys inside know that Ladder 5 "got the roof." As flames nearly rolled over Engine 10, water from the pump, starting at 150 psi but diminishing to about 90 psi by journey's end because of friction loss made its way through the line to the top of the stairs and to the "pipe" in Roland's hands. As soon as he felt the line fill he opened the gate, backed up by Keith and hit the fire with about three hundred gallons a minute. They knocked the visible flames down.

While Engine 8 took care of the water supply, Engine 13 arrived on scene, took another line from the back of Engine 10 and advanced through the rear door to back up Engine 10. Ladder 2 had arrived on scene and started search and rescue operations. They split into two two man teams, entered the smoke filled house, battled their way up three flights of stairs and searched for victims. Engine 8, having established a water supply joined the fight, taking a line through the front door to the second floor.

"Command to ladder 2, I need a status report. I have reports of people inside the third floor apartment."

"Ladder 2 received, starting primary search."

Special hazards arrived and raised ground ladders to the windows on the third floor, giving possibly trapped victims and firefighters a secondary means of egress.

"Engine 10 to command, we've got most of the fire knocked down and confined to a third floor bedroom," came the muffled report.

"Command received."

I watched the drama unfold and silently prayed there were no kids in the house, the specter of a similar scenario from early in my career appeared in my mind through the smoky street and chaos. I never know when disturbing memories will haunt me. The images from that dreadful day years ago were so fresh it felt as though I was reliving the horrific experience all over.

That day, a Sunday at 3:10 in the afternoon, I sat playing cards with the guys from Branch Avenue. I had been detailed to Rescue 3 for the day and was bored. Being new and eager to fight fire I said, "A little fire around here would be nice." I got my wish. Seconds later the bell tipped alerting us to a house fire. The house was located diagonally across the street from the Admiral Street fire station, about five miles away from us. A mother had left her kids at home with a young babysitter while she went out for a drink. The babysitter left shortly after the mother, looking for fun, thinking the kids were sleeping. They weren't. The gang from Branch Avenue roared out of the station toward the fire, Engine 2 in the lead, Ladder 7 close behind, me driving Rescue 3 and the Chief behind us. We all had a job to do and looked forward to the excitement and challenge fires provide. Sometimes, the best part of the fire is responding to the scene. Engine 12 and Ladder 3 from the Admiral Street Station had already begun the battle. We waited to hear what waited as we roared toward the scene.

The radio confirmed, "Code Red!" We stepped it up.

As soon as we arrived, a firefighter ran out of the house, his mask still covering his face, pass device blaring, indicating that his airpack was nearly empty. In his arms he carried a smoldering, unconscious child. Seconds later, another firefighter came out of the building with another child. We placed both kids on the stretcher and broke for the rescue, one-hundred feet away.

Neither child had a pulse or was breathing. We attempted CPR. The protective gloves that I wore melted to one of the babies when I attempted compressions. The other child's lungs were so badly burned we were unable to get air into them. Six of us, with Captain Dave Raymond in charge rode to the trauma room with two dead, smoldering kids. Dave probably knew they were gone but did his best keeping us busy in the lifesaving efforts, knowing the emotional carnage that was to follow. Maybe we worked so hard trying to keep ourselves sane. We arrived at the trauma room and handed our tiny patients over to the trauma teams. They were pronounced dead soon after. Captain Raymond stood in the doorway as the babies were covered with sheets. I stood alone, further down trauma alley. I watched as he finally let go, his body slumped, his head hung low, one hand ran through his hair and the other wiped tears from his face. He slid down the wall stopping in the same spot I would be in years later, numb from watching a college kid fall eighty feet to his death. Thank God there is a floor at the bottom of the wall to catch us when we're falling.

I will never forget the feel of tender young flesh melting into my own. The smell of their burned skin haunted me after the flames were doused. The pungent scent lingered for weeks, every time my hands drew near my face I inhaled the essence of those two suffering kids. I'll never forget them, their names, and their lives. I read all of the news stories that followed the tragedy. I felt as though I knew them, though all I really knew was the anguish they felt as the fire one of them accidentally started by playing with matches burned their tiny bodies. Their faces were frozen with fear, their last expression reflecting the horror of their final minutes. They ran away from the fire that grew bigger than they could ever have imagined, into a back bedroom and under a bed. The firefighters found them under a mattress, much too late.

Dave held a bunch of new firefighters together during that frantic rush to the hospital, made us feel as though we made a difference. Almost everybody on the scene of that fire would eventually receive a Department Commendation and a medal to pin on their dress uniform at Medals Night in April honoring the firefighters who performed heroic deeds the previous year. One guy who didn't get a medal that day is, in my opinion the one who deserved it most. Captain Raymond. The official reason for the slight was that he didn't put his life in jeopardy attempting a rescue. The real reason is that guys that ride the rescues don't get much respect from their fellow firefighters. Captain Raymond's actions that day have stayed with me through my career, and I only hope I have handled myself as well.

The next day, another hero of mine from that terrible day helped put things into perspective. I was in the station, blaming myself for the disaster. Chief Ronny Moura, grizzled veteran firefighter and all around tough guy overheard me say, "I'll never wish for another fire."

Chief Moura stopped in his tracks and said, voice deep and scratchy from eating smoke for decades, "kid, any firefighter worth half a shit wants fires. Quit crying and get off the fucking cross, we need the wood!" then walked away. That fact that Chief Moura thought I was worth half a shit made my night. Eventually I got off the cross and waited for wood to burn again, but never with the same passion.

The report from Ladder 2 brought me back.

"Ladder 2 to command, primary search negative." There was nobody home. Relief flooded the fireground.

Something else flooded the fireground, soaking me and Mike as we stood outside, waiting for victims that thankfully would never appear.

Captain Healy stood in the second floor window holding a charged line. He looked right at us and said, "sorry, didn't see you," blasted us again then pulled the line through the window, looking like the cat who ate the canary. The water fight was over. There was always next year.

TWENTY-THREE

"Engine 11 with a Cranston rescue; respond to 111 Resevior Avenue for a man with ten days of diarrhea."

"Rescue 1 clearing the fire, we'll handle."

"Roger Rescue 1, Engine 11 disregard, we'll cancel Cranston."

With one radio transmission I've made a lot of friends. Cranston rescues hate coming to Providence. The rescue crews from surrounding communities think the Providence rescues hang around all day waiting for the good stuff, shootings, stabbings, electrocutions and the like and hide when the shitty runs come in. They are only partly right.

Run 22 @ 1543 hrs. (3:43 p.m.)

"I love these runs," said Mike as we drove to our destination.

"We've been running like crazy." I responded.

"I hope we don't get the run around."

"Let's run right over there."

"Time could be running out."

"We've had a lot of runs today."

"We've had the run of the city."

"I hope we don't run out of gas."

"This is my kind of run." Mike finished the absurd conversation. I let him get the last word, not because I'm a nice guy, but I ran out of comebacks.

A man in his forties waited outside. He had a door at the top of ten cement steps propped open.

"Hey guys, thanks for getting here so quick. It's my father, he's been throwing up and having diarrhea for ten days. I'm worried he's getting dehydrated. What's up with you guys," he asked. "Your soaked."

"We don't want to get dehydrated so we soak ourselves with water every hour," said Mike. I grinned and shook my head.

"Where is he?" I asked.

"Right over here," he said and led us into their home. The kitchen was clean but cluttered with paperwork. Pictures of Red Sox and Bruins players decorated the walls. A signed photo of Roger Clemens posing with the man who met us at the door was held to the refrigerator door with a banana magnet.

"Hey," the man said, looking at me like he knew me, "you could be Roger Clemens's brother. You look just like him."

"Really?" I asked. Nobody ever said that to me before.

"No way," said Mike, shaking his head.

"No, really," the man continued. "I met Roger at the Marriott a couple of years ago. I'm telling you, you could be his twin."

I'm not sure if this is a good thing or not.

The patient sat in a recliner in a room just off the kitchen. He looked awful, his skin the grey of the coldest sky of winter yet sweat formed on his forehead giving the illusion of transparency on his seasoned face. His eyes were surrounded with black circles, three layers deep. He was wiped out.

"Mike, get the chair."

Mike was gone before I finished saying it. One look at the man told us he wouldn't be walking to the truck.

"How are you feeling?" I asked him.

"Awfully weak." He responded, tired. "I've been vomiting with diarrhea for ten days now. I can't stop. He was apologetic, as though his condition was his own fault.

"Let's get you to the hospital then, you look terrible," I said.

"His doctors are at Fatima. Any chance you could take him there?" the son asked.

Fatima is the furthest hospital from us. With rush hour traffic to contend with the trip will take fifteen minutes. His condition wasn't life threatening. Rhode Island Hospital was a nut house with a six-hour wait, and more importantly, I liked these guys. I don't have to take people to the hospital of their choice, but I wanted to help them out.

"No problem," I said. I would have taken this guy to Florida. I really don't know why, but sometimes I instantly like people.

"Thanks, we really appreciate it," said the son.

"Pop, these guys are going to take care of you, I'll meet you at the hospital later."

"Make sure you lock up," the older man said to his son as we wheeled him out the same door he had walked out of thousands of times and carried him to the rescue. How humbling old age can be. After a quick set of vital signs, we were on our way.

"How long have you lived in that house?" I asked him.

"Be fifty years next week. There's five bedrooms upstairs. Me and my wife would have celebrated our fiftieth anniversary if she hadn't died a couple of years ago. We bought the house for seven thousand dollars! Can you believe that! I could sell it tomorrow for two hundred thousand." His voice picked up steam as he went on.

"More than that, I bet. The place is beautiful."

"You should have seen it when my wife was alive. Women have a way with those kind of things." He had a far away look in his eyes as he reminisced. I wonder what he's thinking.

"Do you live there alone?" I asked.

"No, my boy lives with me. He's a great kid. I don't know what I'd do without him."

"From the look of him, he feels the same way about you."

"We're lucky to have each other. He looks out for me, and I give him something to do."

A teamster's baseball cap sat proudly on Harry's head. He was a big man in his day. Though his shoulders were hunched and he had shrunk with age, he still exuded a certain power. The days of vomiting and diarrhea hadn't taken the sparkle from his eye when he talked about the past and his family. This was a good, hard working man, the kind that I aspire to be, and hope I am. He took care of his family to the best of his ability, "done his damndest," provided a beautiful home and lived a good life. These things were obvious to anybody fortunate enough to be in his presence. I as glad I went in service and took this run.

"What kind of work did you do with the teamsters?" I asked.

"I started driving truck, then went on to manage the warehouse at the print works. Thirty men worked for me back then. I don't think the warehouse is even in operation now, all the work is overseas."

My father started his career after the war with the phone company as a janitor. He stayed with the company until he died at sixty-one. He was an engineer with thirty or more people working for him.

"You're right. It's a shame what's happened to the country."

"It still is the best country on earth." He said the words simply, without any unnecessary embellishment.

On impulse I asked Harry, "Were you in the war?"

I like to ask people his age what they did during World War II. I am amazed at the different answers I get. Some served in the armed forces, others stayed stateside and helped in their own way. I wonder how it feels to be of an age eligible to have fought in that war and answer people of my generation's questions. Are they decorated war heroes? Do they feel shame if they weren't heroic fighting men? Were they proud that they didn't participate?

"Army. Pacific for three years."

"How was it?" I asked.

"Terrible."

He wasn't upset but obviously didn't want to talk about it. I had the feeling that if he did we would be in California before his story was through.

"Thank you for your service to the country." I was barely able to get the words out, my voice choked up. I don't know why I got so emotional, but I always have. These old geezers bring it out. Some day I'll be in their shoes and hope I have half of Harry's dignity.

I felt the truck stop and knew we had arrived. Our Lady of Fatima Hospital is actually in North Providence, a city separate from Providence. It is confusing, South Providence is part of the City of Providence, but North Providence and East Providence are not. They each have their own government and services. For such a small state, Rhode Island is very confusing. West Providence doesn't exist, but we do have the West End, a part of Providence. The East Side is also part of Providence, but don't confuse that with East Providence. There are a lot of politicians in such a small area.

"What's all the chatter back here? I'm getting an earache." Mike said while opening the rear doors of the rescue. He has a way with words.

We brought Harry into the hospital by way of the rescue doors. One indication that we were not in the inner city anymore was the sign asking the rescue drivers to turn off their engines. It read,

"Due to the close proximity of the patients to the ambulance door, we kindly ask the ambulance drivers to turn off their engines before leaving their vehicles. Thank you so much for your cooperation."

I always got a chuckle from the sign when thinking of the security guards at Rhode Island Hospital telling the drivers the same thing, only not so kindly. *"Turn off the fucking engine,"* is more like it.

I said goodbye to Harry. People come into my life and leave too quickly. Some hang around for a while in my mind; others are forgotten as soon as they leave the truck. Harry will be around for a very long time.

It seemed like an eternity since I was last here but it was only last night. I took a look around the treatment area for the lady from Sandringham Avenue but she was nowhere to be found. She was probably admitted to one of the rooms. I hoped so.

TWENTY-FOUR

"Those guys were pretty cool," said Mike as we drove around the back of Fatima, through the parking lot brimming with parked cars and onto the road toward home. Every hospital in the area was full of patients. One comes, another leaves. One lives, one dies. There must be a plan; there has to be.

"Yeah, they were. I hope the old guy is all right." Mike missed much of my conversation with Harry, and I'm not sure he would be interested. "Do you think I look like Roger Clemens?"

"No way. He was sucking up trying to get you to take his father to Fatima."

"You think so?"

"No doubt about it." Mike drives while I doze in the officer's seat. Rank has its privileges.

Rush hour traffic was unbearable. The trip back to our district from Fatima is about seven miles long. At this time of day it normally takes half an hour to get back to quarters. Not today. The radio was tuned to WBRU, Brown University's excellent FM station. I've been listening to them for thirty years, although lately the music doesn't do it for me. At one time I liked most of what they played, now I only find a small percentage fits my taste. I'm sure it has nothing to do with the number of birthday's I have endured.

"Hey, the Dropkick Murphy's!" I said while turning up the volume and waking from my nap. The guys in the band are regular Joe's from Boston who love traditional Irish music. They combined that with Punk and Hard Rock to create a heavenly sound, for those so inclined. Anybody that can incorporate bagpipes into a punk rock band has my loyal following. They are on the verge of making it big, but I don't think that is what motivates them. There is a joy and edge to their music that I haven't heard in years.

I play hockey for the Providence Fire Department's team. We play in a league against other fire departments. For the past ten years, Anthony Lancelotti, the guy who runs the league, has organized a charity tournament involving firefighter and police teams from all over the region. As part of the festivities, he holds a steak fry and raffle at the end of the tournament, all proceeds going to charity. I sent an e-mail to the band in January asking for some help with the tournament, hoping for a CD or something to use in the raffle. The band came through with CD's, an autographed picture with all the band members, some tour shirts and some hockey jerseys. They went so far as to offer their services on the ice, but scheduling conflicts negated that.

"Isn't this the band you saw last week at Lupo's?"

"Same one." The fire department requires a firefighter to be on premises at events of more than one-thousand people. I worked the night of the concert.

"The place was packed, people milling about having a good time and waiting for the band. The crowd started chanting; 'Lets go Murphy's, Lets go Murphy's. Then the lights went down with nothing but a spotlight focusing on a bagpiper in the middle of the stage in full Scottish regalia. He played a nice traditional tune; the people really got into it. When the song was over, the rest of the stage lights came on, the Dropkick Murphy's took the stage and began to play. The crowd was moshing, the band was rocking, and then the piper put down his pipes and dove into the crowd for some surfing. The place went wild. It was the greatest thing I've ever seen," I told Mike, but he didn't seem impressed.

"You're a little old for the mosh pit don't you think?" he said, shaking his head. He is more of a classic hard rock guy.

"I invented the mosh pit. We were slam dancing to the Ramones before most of the kids in the crowd were even born."

"Like I said, a little old for the mosh pit."

I'll never understand the younger generation.

"You're too old to be playing hockey too."

"I feel too old to be doing much of anything. I don't know if it's the job or Father Time, but the last few years have really taken their toll. But I'll still kick your ass." I said as we closed in on South Providence.

"Getting old," Mike said, ignoring me. "At least I have something to look forward to."

I picked up the mike and threw myself to the wolves.

"Rescue 1 is in service."

"Roger Rescue 1, respond to 1035 Broad Street for an intoxicated male."

Run 23 @ 1615 hrs. (4:15 p.m.)

"No rest for the wicked," said Mike. I just shook my head. We never made it to the repair shop, were running low on fuel and I still hadn't picked up the manicotti.

"Rescue 1 responding."

The lights and sirens were on. Mike drove while I dozed. It seemed seconds later we were stopped in front of 1035 Broad Street. A man was lying in the parking lot of the liquor store, twitching. People went about their business without missing a beat. Mike and I gloved up and got him.

"Leroy!" said Mike as if greeting an old friend. Leroy said nothing, just continued twitching.

"We're not carrying you, Leroy so get up." I said, crossing my arms and standing over our patient.

"I'm having a seizure." Leroy croaked, shaking on the filthy pavement. "Please, take me to Miriam."

All of the drunks want to go to Miriam. The staff there doesn't deal with them as often as the people at Rhode Island Hospital; subsequently they are treated better. It's not that they don't get good care at Rhode Island, Miriam just doesn't see them every day and have more patience. They've yet to wear out their welcome.

"All right, walk to the truck and we'll take you to Miriam." Mike said convincingly.

"You're lyin. You're gonna take me to Rhode Island. I am beyond reproach motherfucker! Take me to Miriam," roared Leroy, much like a king giving orders to his servants.

"Leroy," I said reproachfully. "You know the rules."

There aren't any rules, but I like to pretend there are.

"They beat me up at Rhode Island," he says.

Mike put things into perspective. "They don't take your bullshit is more like it."

"That is because, I am beyond reproach! Rock and Roll, lose control!" he shouted. The party is over for him and he knows it. He planned for his daily drinking binge to end this way. When he had enough, he faked a seizure, some dummy with a cell phone called it in and he waited for us to take him to the hospital.

He got up, dusted himself off and made his way to the truck. He had feces running down the back of his pants. Mike saw it and sped toward the truck to put down a barrier sheet between the bench seat and Leroy.

Of all the homeless alcoholics that I have dealt with over the years, Leroy is the one I think has the best chance of getting sober. The rest of the rescue guys think I'm nuts, but I think he has the potential. Every now and then he drops out of sight for a few weeks. The story is that he has a wife who lets him stay with her only when he is not drinking. When I don't see him I hope he is drying out at his wife's house.

The seizure game was over and Leroy sat in the rescue pleading with me to take him to Miriam. Rhode Island Hospital doesn't play games with the drunks. We bring them to the triage area where their vital signs are taken, then their alcohol level assessed. If they respond to verbal stimuli they are off to the "tanks" where they are monitored until sobering up. If they are unresponsive they're taken to a trauma room and given a thorough work-up. This costs the taxpayers thousands of dollars. When their blood alcohol level reaches an acceptable level they are released. If, as is Leroy's case today, they need to be cleaned up, the emergency room technicians have to do it. They are stripped and taken to a de-con shower and treated like contaminated victims from a haz-mat incident. Newcomers are offered counseling. The regulars have been counseled so many times the medical community has given up. They are on their own; all attempts of rehabilitation have failed. If they act up during their stay, security is on them quick. Restraints are common and necessary. The regulars like Darryl and Leroy don't need to be restrained too often, but when they get out of line the guards are not shy or gentle.

I was in the back of the rescue sitting in the captain's chair filling out the state form while Leroy sat on the bench seat, looking miserable. I didn't have to ask him any questions; I know the answers. His name, date of birth, past medical history, medicine taken, and allergies to medicine all flew from the tip of my pen with me barely guiding it.

"When are you going to smarten up?" I asked him.

"I'm an alcoholic," is his response, as if that explains everything.

"So what?"

"I need help."

"You need to quit drinking."

"You don't know what it's like."

"Yes I do."

I said it without being condescending and it takes Leroy by surprise. He looked at me and asked with a smirk, "What does a rich white boy know about anything."

"I know that if I don't drink and go to meetings I have a good life. If I drink, I'll be an asshole like you."

Leroy closes his eyes and gives in to his fate. Every alcoholic who wants to get sober knows the truth is, we're victims to a terrible disease. Some recover, most don't. The only difference between these bums and me is that I don't drink. I was there once, and could be again. All it takes is one. As long as I keep things in perspective, I'll be all right.

TWENTY-FIVE

"What are you up to tonight?" I asked Mike once we were rid of Leroy.

"Painting Easter Eggs. Henry's waiting for the Easter Bunny."

"What about Sammy?"

"He doesn't believe in the Easter Bunny."

"He's a month old."

"I told you he was smart."

We couldn't wait to get home. Mike's wife, Amy would have three boys to baby-sit when he got there. I could only imagine the fun that must go on at their house. Mike is truly insane. His boys will probably follow in his footsteps.

We had dispatched Leroy. He'd be released later that night and go through the routine again. I would be home and away from the nonsense.

"Let's get some fuel and call it a day. We'll fix the thing that holds the stretcher tomorrow."

"Good thinking. This will keep us out of service until we get relieved."

"What do you think, this is my first day?" I asked. Mike gives me one of his thousands of looks and drives. I had been running non-stop since yesterday at seven in the morning. I was tired, but it was a good tired. I managed just enough sleep throughout the two days to keep me going. Thirty-four hours goes fast when working at a busy pace. There are periods during that time that it feels like the runs will never end, but every week I get through it.

Sometimes, I think of my days in the image of an hourglass. As the sands run through from top to bottom so does my shift. When it is through, I'll have some time off, and then I'll turn the glass over and start again.

I had responded to twenty-three emergency calls since reporting for duty yesterday. Some people needed help, some thought they needed help, and some needed a ride or somebody to talk to.

The portable radio is like a monkey on my back. When my relief came in, I'd finally be rid of it. Although it takes time to relax after days being in a state of readiness, it is imperative that I do so. Taking the job home is a big mistake. I have learned to distance myself from the department when I'm not there. Some guys can't get enough of it; I prefer to leave it behind. I go so far as to not wear anything blue during my time off.

The fuel pumps are located near the waterfront a few blocks from the fire station. Mike pulled the rescue up to the pump, got out and began fueling. The truck takes around thirty gallons of diesel to fill, Mike put twenty-six into the tank. We were almost dry. Before we left the fueling station the radio crackles.

"Engine 13 a still alarm, a rescue run."

"Shit, we're going to have to take that." I said. I'm so close to the end I can see the finish line. My plan to get out of the city on time was foiled again. One more wouldn't kill me. I keyed the mike.

"Rescue 1, clearing the pumps."

Run 24 @ 1644 hrs. (4:45 p.m.)

"Roger Rescue 1, respond to 1212 Allens Ave for a woman feeling ill."

"Rescue 1 responding."

This sounded like another taxi ride to the hospital. There's nothing wrong with a nice easy run to finish things up. The trip to the ill woman's home took about three minutes; she walked out of her house as soon as we pulled in front toward to the rescue.

"I'm in pain," she informed us. I got out and opened the side door.

She was fifty and told me that she has been living with pain for years and nobody could help her. Her private doctors had prescribed painkillers but they didn't work. Every move she made was accentuated with grunts and groans and the look on her face was pure agony as she climbed the two steps into the truck. Another nut.

"I'm going to get your vital signs," Mike informed her and placed the blood pressure cuff over her upper left arm. The machine is automatic; Mike pressed a button and the cuff began to inflate.

"It hurts!" our patient yelled as the cuff tightened.

"It only hurts for a second then begins to deflate." I told her, a little impatiently. I was out of compassion for the day.

It appeared that she endured a Chinese water torture during the process. I was tempted to start an IV with a large bore needle just to be mean, but the angel on my left shoulder overruled the devil on my right.

Her vital signs were normal, the painful procedure over. We headed back to Rhode Island Hospital, hopefully for the last time today. My patient, Celeste sat on the bench seat. I looked at her from the captain's chair.

"Can you work with all of the pain?" I asked to pass the time.

"I'm an artist so I work a lot from my house. I also have a studio in Warwick. It's hard to be creative when living with so much pain," she winced.

"What is the cause of all the pain?" I asked. I really wanted to know if she had Lyme disease of something similar, had an accident or if she is a nut.

"No cause, just something I have to endure."

She didn't look like a nut, or act like one. People are so alike, yet so different. We will never know how it feels to be inside another person's mind or body. A minor irritation to one person is major pain to another. We are wired differently, I figured.

"What is the emergency room going to do for you?" I asked.

"Help me."

"How?"

"With medication." That settled that. She is going to alleviate her pain. Why she needed a rescue to get her there is beyond me. Sitting inside her purse, on top is a fantasy/science fiction novel that I read years ago.

"Do you like the book?" I asked. She followed the direction of my gaze with her eyes.

"Oh, that. The story is all right, but I really like the cover art. This is what I do," she picked the book up and showed me the cover.

"You did that?" I asked.

"Not this one, but I've done a lot of similar things. I really love the Tolkien stories. I've done some murals for those books."

"Really? What is your favorite subject to paint?" Suddenly, I was wide awake. I grew up reading the Hobbit and The Lord of the Rings. I've read all of the books dozens of times. The movie versions are popular now, but you can't beat a good book.

"I painted the mirror of Galadriel, Treebeard and The Black Rider's at Bern. The originals are at my studio."

"They must be worth a small fortune." I said. She laughed, then grimaced and replied whimsically, "You would be surprised at how small a fortune they are worth."

"That's too bad. Creativity should be worth more than it is." I said.

"It's not all about the money. I have a good life and I love my art. I just hate living in pain."

"Where is your studio?"

Celeste told me where she worked and I promised to stop by. I looked forward to seeing her work. No matter how long I do this job I seem to never learn the simplest things. Never judge a book by its cover is one of those simple sayings that I should pay closer attention to. Another fascinating person had just graced the inside of the rescue, yet I was ready to dismiss her without a second thought. I have a privilege that must never be taken for granted. People let me into their homes, share with me their secrets and trust me with their lives. When I think of the enormity of that I am overwhelmed.

For the day's last time, I felt the truck make the turn into the rescue bay at Rhode Island Hospital, the bump at the end of the driveway shaking the truck right on cue. Mike turned and backed into the bay. I helped Celeste out of the side door and we walked into the triage area together. There was a break in the action, the night shift had taken over. Tarah was standing at the desk, saw us, punched her report into the time clock and asked, "What have you got?"

"Fifty year old female, complaining of pain all over, ongoing problem for years, no trauma or diagnosis, takes pain medication with no allergies to meds, vitals stable, ambulated to the truck, sign here."

"Long shift?" asked Tarah.

"Is it that obvious?"

"We usually can't get rid of you, now you can't wait to leave." She said and signed my report.

"See you tomorrow," I said goodbye to Celeste and walked back to the truck. The people we deal with at the hospital see a lot of us. We tend to hang around there between runs and sometimes wear out our welcome.

This was definitely it. The ride back to quarters took five minutes. Mark was waiting at the station. I removed the portable radio from my belt and passed it over to him. I'm relieved. The torch had been passed again.

EPILOGUE

9:38

My clock doesn't tell me if it is morning or night. I remember coming home, trying to stay awake, failing. I want to have a normal life, spend time with my wife and kids, but I can't. Maybe someday.

There is no light coming from the spaces between the window shades. Night. I've been asleep for two hours. Cheryl probably has dinner in the oven, hoping that I'll join her. I usually do. She'll go hungry waiting for me to come downstairs. It is an effort to be pleasant, but she deserves that. Sometimes I fail and she puts me back to bed where I sleep on and off until morning. I'm going to stay awake tonight, at least until eleven.

The fight we had about the forgotten manicotti is over, I think. I'll pick it up tomorrow

when I go back to work. In a few hours I'll start another marathon shift, then have a few days off.

My corner of the world, Providence, is a little better off because of the work I do. It is

a small contribution in the big scheme of things, but I find satisfaction in that. The people I meet and help are truly players on the worlds stage. Each individual has a part, some seemingly insignificant yet vital, others apparently enormous yet trivial.

Firefighters die saving people from burning buildings and are given a heroes farewell, thousands attending the funeral, thousands more watching on television. The people that weren't saved are laid to rest in relative anonymity. Murderers walk free, their victims gone forever. Young people are killed in car accidents by drunken drivers who continue to drink and drive. Kids fall off of dorm roofs to their untimely death, never reaching their potential as their families ponder what could have been.

Tomorrow begins another day. How many lives will be changed forever? Will it be my turn? I guess I'm going to find out.

RESCUE 1

RESPONDING

"Never in the history of human conflict, has so much been owed by so many, to so few."

—Winston S. Churchill

For Kellie and John

FORWARD

I am the rescue guy. People call me during their worst moments. When things go badly I take them in, patch their wounds, calm their fears and help them breathe. I stop their bleeding and keep them alive. At least I try. My time with them is short, usually ten minutes or less. In that period of time I learn a lot, and sometimes teach a little, but always leave with a better understanding of the human condition.

They think I help them, and I do to some degree, but more often than not it is they who help me. Every person who crosses my path teaches me a little more about things, some great, others small, but always something.

THE BEGINNING

Daylight. The blinds obscure sun's rays, but the dawn of a new day is impossible to hide. I think it's about nine. If that is true, I've been out for ten hours. From the look of the covers, I haven't moved much. There's nothing like a thirty-four hour shift to put you into death sleep.

Last night, Cheryl made dinner for us, I remember eating, forcing myself to stay awake. I failed miserably at pleasantry; she must have put me back to bed after a little while. I tried to stay up when I got home but fell asleep sitting on the couch. I snored for a few hours according to all reports, but I'm sure the nature of the noises emanating from me is grossly exaggerated.

For five years I've worked the overtime between shifts making a great schedule nearly impossible. Rather than two ten hour days followed with two fourteen hour nights, I now do two marathons, a thirty-four, twenty-four off followed by a thirty-eight. I'm headed for the thirty-eight in a few hours.

Why?

It started as a challenge. I enjoyed the chaos, the sleep deprivation, pushing my mind and body to the extreme, yet still performing. I think it was my ego that started the whole thing; I did it because I could. It's difficult, and not many thrive, but I was one of the few that did. Or so I thought. It's a simple thing to go to work, put everything else away and worry about only yourself. It has taken a while, but slowly I've learned that without everybody else, myself just ain't that great.

Now, I'm stuck with the overtime. Circumstances change, needs arise, one thing leads to another and before you know it what once was a challenge becomes business as usual.

Nobody in bed with me, no cats, no dogs, no wife. Alone again. You get used to it. I've got Friday and Saturday night in the city to look forward to, and Saturday all day as a bonus. Thirty-eight straight, and I'm going in with one eye open. And leaving my family alone again. Easter Sunday is coming, lots to do, not enough time to do it. As the day approaches the tension mounts. I know that somehow we'll pull it all together, and we'll have our holiday, and a great dinner, and somehow the manicotti will appear along with the ham and potato croquettes. I just hope I'm awake to enjoy it.

You take all of your experience and memories with you on every call. What we present is the culmination of every one. The learning never stops, the growing never ends. My twenty-four hours is up, time to get back at it.

PART I

FRIDAY NIGHT

1630 hrs. (4:30 p.m.)

"Bye, babe, see you in a couple of days."
"Be careful."
I smile and walk out the door. "Be careful" is the last thing I like to hear before heading into the city. It's been that way going on sixteen years now. Maybe I'm superstitious, but I worry if I don't hear those words.

My bag is filled with the necessities; a few changes of clothes, a big bag of peanut M&M's, a book, a few magazines and the usual assortment of overnight things. I hang my spare uniform, still warm from the iron and smelling faintly of starch onto the hook in the backseat, open the door and get in. With any luck in forty hours I'll be home again, worn out but satisfied, with four days of peace and quiet ahead.

I wave to Brittany as she speeds past me as I pull onto the pavement. "Slow down," I say out loud to the empty car. It's chilly, she's wearing a winter hat, the kind that ties on the bottom and has earflaps to keep you warm. She doesn't have a care in the world, and that makes me happy. I long for those days but for me they are gone forever. That's probably a good thing, without worries we would have no experience of things to worry about and go through life thinking everything is fair and safe. It's not, but at least for my kids it will be for a little while longer.

Traffic is slow and heavy, the streets and roads full of people coming home after a long week at work. As I approach Providence the traffic clears a little, at least on my side of the road. Most people are leaving the city. I'm going in.

About 180,000 people officially live in Providence, a lot more if you count the undocumented immigrants. Thousands more commute from the neighboring cities and towns, spend their time in the Capitol City then leave for their suburban retreats. I turn on the radio and check in on the local talk shows. Nothing new, the same talk of high taxes, corrupt politicians, failing schools and on and on. Today, there is no mention of the firefighters, who have been a hot topic lately. The FM dial is a little more interesting, Blue Sky by the Allman Brothers sticks, I take my finger off the seek button and settle in.

It's staying light later now, as winter loosens its icy grasp on Rhode Island. Loosens, but doesn't let go.

I like to drive. I find the routine, mechanical movements relaxing. I know the road to work so well the car could drive itself. It gives me time to think. An incident from last week comes to mind, though I try to push it away.

It had been quiet for about an hour, the only sounds I could hear came from the open window of my office as the late night bar crowd straggled past the station on their way home. A few drunken shouts, tires squealing, bottles breaking on the pavement as people cleared out their pre-club empties before heading home. I turned the portable off, hoping to sneak a few hours sleep in before the next run. It had been a long shift, thirty or so calls so far with six hours to go. At one time most of my time was spent being on call, now, it seems all of my time is spent on calls. Almost, but not all. I hit the bunk and was out cold before my head touched the pillow.

0230 hrs (2:30 a.m.)

"*Rescue 5 and Ladder 4, Respond to 1 Providence Place for a woman who has fallen.*"

Ladder 4 was out of the building before I made it to the rescue. Tim waited for me, the engine running. He saw me from the rear view mirrors and turned the engine over. The piercing wail from the truck's siren scattered the people lingering in front of the station as we rolled pat them, closing the overhead door behind us. As we passed Water Place Park, the officer of Ladder 4 gave his report.

"*Ladder 4 to Rescue 5, twenty-five year old female, fell approximately forty feet, massive head injury.*"

"*Rescue 5, received.*"

I hung the mike back in it's cradle and put on some gloves. One Providence Place is an enormous shopping mall located in Downtown Providence. The building takes up four blocks of real estate, big enough to warrant its own zip code. Tim made his approach, stopping behind the ladder truck, in front of the north entryway. Most of the stores were closed at this hour. A movie theater and restaurant occupied the upper levels and stayed open late. We loaded the stretcher with a long spine board and med bag and made our way into the mall. A lone security guard stood outside the entrance. I asked if he knew anything about the incident.

"*Somebody fell.*"

We walked past him, up the ramp toward the elevators. The mall is a confusing place when shopping, worse when seconds count. Overlooking the balcony next to the elevators I saw the guys from Ladder 4 two floors

below me, working on a young woman. A dark shadow outlined her head.
We walked into the elevator car, stopped and looked at the buttons.

"LL, 1, 1M, GF, 2, 2M, 3L, 3, 4."

"Which floor?" I asked Tim.

"First."

I hit the 1 button and slammed my fist into the panel when the elevator started going up. I was a little more tense than I thought. The elevator wouldn't stop until it made it to the first floor no matter how many times I pushed the LL button. After an eternity it did stop, then reverse direction. At 1M the elevator stopped again, the doors opening to an empty floor. Gaining control of my emotions I pushed LL and felt the box begin its decent, agonizingly slow. Finally, the doors opened on the proper floor.

John Morgan, a truck mate of mine from another part of my career held the girl's head in his hands while I tried to apply a cervical collar.

"It's soft," he said, cradling the back of her head while I wrapped the hard plastic around her neck. I reached around back and felt the crushed skull, like jelly where there should have been bone. I checked her pupils, shining light into her eyes hoping to see a reaction. There was a reaction, though not in her eyes. A sick feeling started in the middle of my chest and worked its way through my body. "She's my daughter's age," I said out loud.

"Fixed and dilated." I stood and stepped back while the crew from Ladder 4 and Tim immobilized her, assisted ventilations and put her on the stretcher. They had all been around long enough to know the girl's chances for survival were none and none. Off to the side a young couple and a solitary young man stood watching, ashen faced.

"Will she be all right?" asked the young guy who stood alone.

"We're doing everything we can," I replied, again, knowing that all we could do would never be enough. The girl was gone; the best we could do was keep her heart pumping and hope for a miracle. Somewhere, somebody waiting for a kidney or a liver just hit the lottery. The thought made me sick so I pushed it aside.

"What happened?" I asked.

He pointed up to an area of escalators, three stories above us.

"She fell."

The stretcher was moving now, a group of firefighters pushing the stretcher toward the elevator, bagging and picking up the mess we made with our equipment. We all fit into the elevator. As the doors closed the only thing that remained was a little Spider Man doll, tossed to the side of the floor, and a dark red stain on the mall's new carpet.

"Slow down," I said again, as much to myself as to Brittany. I found out a few days later that the girl had planned on being married next month. She was a single mother and was about to get a degree from a local community college. She was out celebrating her birthday. She won the Spider Man doll at the nightclub where she spent her last night on this earth and planned on giving it to her four-year old son in the morning. I hope somebody picked the doll up from the mall floor and gave it to its rightful owner. Reading the obituary is worse than living through the experience, there is nothing to do but read about the person who died on your watch, and think about what could have been.

The rescue is not in the bay. "D" group is working today, I'll be relieving Tim, who just started his own four day war. Some of the guys from D group are still waiting to be relived and are sitting around the day room with the oncoming shift.

"Hey, Shakespeare!" says Greg, one of the D-group guys as I walk into the room.

"Nice job on that article."

"What article?" I ask. He hands me the morning's Providence Journal, opened to the letters to the editor section. A letter that I sent to the paper was printed in the morning edition. My heart sinks a little when I see my words printed for anybody to read. I wrote the letter in response to increasing criticism firefighters have been getting in the press and the talk shows. Last week, during my days off I was heading to the store to get some lettuce for a salad I was making and happened to turn on the radio. A local Mayor was on the talk radio station I was tuned to and asked the question, "Why should firefighters get full healthcare coverage when millions of Americans can barely afford to get by?" I only tuned into the end of the show but could only imagine the topic. This particular mayor and his fire department have been at odds for years. His city's firefighter contract is due to expire soon and the mayor has taken to the airwaves and editorials to discredit the fire service. As revenue shrinks cities and towns, strapped for cash are desperate to save money, at times recklessly endangering the public by under funding public safety.

I called the talk show when I got home and talked to the host for about ten minutes. I was pleasantly surprised that he let me state my side of the issue, and he seemed genuinely impressed by our side of things. However, when I hung up the phone, I felt I needed to say more. The salad waited and I wrote down my feelings. The letter took me all night to write. Angry callers reacting to the words I had spoken on the radio filled the room from the radio speaker as I typed. I was not a big hit with the audience.

I take the paper from Greg and get a weird feeling as I read my own words:

Dear Editor,

I do not know the salaries of my friends in the private sector. It is not my business to scrutinize their benefit package. I do know that they work as hard as I do making a living. Some of them are doing better, some not as well. We are all getting by.

The struggling economy has made us all aware of our financial vulnerability. As salaries and benefits stagnate, resentment grows. Through the ups and downs, my financial situation remains steady. For years I watched as others reaped the rewards of a strong economy. Nobody noticed or cared about my pay and benefits. My modest income paled in comparison to those in the private sector.

Now, my pay and benefits are front-page news. Cities and towns are facing budget deficits: the unions are to blame. Headlines and letters scream, "The party is over! The bleeding must stop!" If I didn't know better, I would think the state is full of impoverished workers with no benefits at all!

I am a firefighter. I have a good salary, great benefits and an exciting job. I will not apologize for it or willingly give it up. Thirteen years ago I was accepted into the Providence Fire Department's 42nd Training Academy. The competition was fierce; thousands applied for a few positions. I never considered myself better than the thousands that didn't make it. Throughout the rigorous testing procedures it was found that some of us have the potential to be better firefighters than the rest. We were hired; the others went about their lives. I know some great people that did not get hired. They are leading productive lives in other pursuits.

I knew I would never get rich being a firefighter but the benefits provide my family with security. Had I not become a firefighter, I'm sure whatever vocation I chose would provide a good life for my wife and kids. I certainly wouldn't worry about my neighbor's paycheck.

The promise of security and the nature of the job are what draw so many to apply. The public is well served by the men and women that make it through the process. If the pay and benefits were average, the pool of applicants would be smaller, and less qualified people would be responding to the calls for help from the community.

I never ask thanks for the job that I do. I read and hear others in my profession justify our compensation because of our bravery. I disagree. Bravery resides in all of us. I see true courage daily. An eighty-year old woman watching quietly as CPR is performed on her husband shows real bravery. I see from glancing at the pictures on the wall images of their life together. Their kids and grandchildren are proudly displayed. The dinner dishes still dry in the sink. Two easy chairs placed in front of the television. The books and papers they have shared. She maintains her composure as we wheel him for the last time out their door and into the night.

I see teenaged kids playing in the streets where their childhood friends were gunned down. They are streetwise beyond their years. They hang around and look tough. Some carry guns. They didn't choose the life they have. They live in a world of violence and chaos. Somehow, if they are hurt, or shot, or sick and make it to the back of my rescue and we are alone, they become kids again. Nice kids too. To live in their world is brave. To visit it and help when we are called is my job.

At times I bring the job home. Years of experience have provided me with ways to cope with the horrors I witness. My family knows when "something's wrong". Tragedy in other people's lives has a way of making its way into ours. I try not to bring it home and mostly am successful. Unfortunately, some incidents can never be left at work and will be a part of me forever. I never know when I will be called to respond to one of these incidents. I know I can always count on my wife. She watches me walk *out our door, dressed in the uniform never knowing if it will be for the last time. Too many times I have left happy and returned distant. She tells me I die a little after every shift. I think she may be right. Being a firefighter's wife takes bravery, being a firefighter is our duty.*

I am exposed to infectious diseases on a daily basis. My body has been punished countless times battling the fires that burn throughout the city. When I retire, I will have healthcare for life. This knowledge helps when considering if the job is worth the risk. AIDS, the fear of SARS, hepatitis, TB and increasingly violent patients all contribute to my dangerous work environment. I don't think good healthcare is too high a price for the taxpayers to bear.

I am fortunate to have the greatest job in the world. I understand that there are some that are envious - the job is worthy of envy. My profession has enabled me to experience life to the fullest. To perform deeds that help lessen humanity's suffering is priceless. I hope that the people of Providence understand what our contribution is worth.

Sincerely,

Michael Morse, Providence Firefighter

It feels strange exposing my thoughts for the world to read. I'm not sure I like it, but I feel strongly about the issue and felt I had to say what needed to be said. I have opened the door for some serious ridicule from the guys. I hope they don't take it too far.

Tim enters the room as I'm finishing the letter, hands me the radio and simply says,

"You've got a run."

ONE

Friday Night.

I take the portable from Tim and get ready for a long shift. I know that I'll be working overtime tomorrow, which means thirty-eight hours straight. The radio comes alive.

"Rescue 1, Respond to 1044 Broad Street, nature unknown."

"Rescue 1, responding."

"Do you think it's Junior?" Mike asks, as we wheel out of the station and into the South Providence neighborhood.
"Maybe. Might be Darryl."
"Might be somebody having a heart attack."
"You never know."
Junior and Darryl are two of our regular customers who haunt the 1000 block of Broad Street. A lot of homeless people linger in a field at 1035 Broad Street. It is a convenient location; a liquor store is on one corner, a convenience store on the other and a pay

phone across the street. A typical day for these folks consists of panhandling money from the convenience store customers, buying a half pint of cheap vodka at the liquor store, drinking it, then stumbling across the street to the pay phone and calling 911 for a ride to the emergency room because they are intoxicated. It drives me crazy that they get away with it, but it works for guys like Darryl and Junior. These guys are survivors, whatever works.

The usual suspects are lined up on a bench next to the liquor store. Five or six people have gathered there, Junior and Darryl among them. Mike stops the rescue, I lower the window and ask, "who's going?"

"We're all set," says somebody from the crowd.

"Over there," says Junior, pointing across the street.

A man in his forties stands outside a storefront clutching his chest, another man helping him stand. We open the back doors of the rescue, grab the stretcher and cross the busy street, dodging cars along the way.

"What's going on?" Mike asks the men.

"His chest hurts," answers the one who is helping the patient stand. We lay him on our stretcher and cross back to the rescue. Junior stumbles to his feet and opens the rear door of the rescue for us.

"Thanks, Junior," I say to him as we lift the stretcher.

"You're my boy, right," he says, extending his hand to shake. I take the offering then pat him on the back and step inside.

"I'm you're boy, Junior," I say and close the doors.

Our patient is around my age, healthy looking and in obvious pain. He clutches his chest and looks around the rescue, frantic, while we get to work.

"What happened," I ask him. He doesn't answer.

"He doesn't speak English," says his friend.

"Do you know what happened?" I ask the other guy.

"We were working in the store," he says, pointing across the street at an empty storefront. "Ramon was sitting on the floor doing paperwork. Suddenly he grabbed his chest and said he couldn't breathe."

"What was he doing right before this happened?" I ask as Mike gets the leads ready. I'm filling the reservoir of a non-rebreather, getting ready to put the mask over the patient's face. Supplemental oxygen is basic protocol but incredibly helpful to a person having a heart attack.

"We are getting ready to open a barber shop. Just moving boxes and things."

I spent months in EMT cardiac school learning how to analyze different rhythms and their underlying cause. We practiced identifying and interpreting everything from a normal sinus rhythm, premature atrial contractions, paroxysmal supraventricular tachycardia, atrial fibrillation, junctional rhythms, PVC's, V-tack, asystole and many more. Mike has finished connecting the leads, runs a strip and hands it to me. I look it over, analyze the p-wave, QRS complex and elevated t-waves and give my diagnosis to Mike.

"He's fucked."

I've narrowed all of the rhythms I learned in school down to two. Fucked and Not Fucked. This guy is fucked. ST elevations mean a myocardial infarction, or death of the heart muscle. Every second we spend on the street means loss of that heart muscle. "Get an IV and go," I say to Mike who has already started looking for a vein. I give the patient four baby aspirin to chew or swallow, then a nitroglycerine tablet to place under his tongue. Oxygen, EKG, Aspirin, IV, Nitro and Go is the best course of action here; we finish our tasks and are moving in less than five minutes.

Rhode Island Hospital is only two and a half miles away. I pick up the phone and let them know we're coming in.

"Rhode Island ER," answers Gary from the triage desk.

"Providence Rescue 1, forty year old male, possible heart, elevated ST's, pulsox 88 on room air, 180/110, IV established, 10 liters 02 by mask, aspirin and nitro on board, ETA two minutes."

"See you in two."

I get the patient's information from his friend and business partner during the short trip to the ER. Both are recent immigrants who plan to open a barbershop on Broad Street. My patient is holding on, the nitro and oxygen helping immediately. Mike backs into the rescue bay and opens the rear doors and we wheel him in.

Gary waits at the door and leads us to one of the trauma rooms. A medical team is in place, another IV started, a 12-lead EKG run and meds administered through our IV line. Gary signs my report and we back out of the room, letting the best medical team anywhere take over his care. Ramon's friend waits outside the trauma room. He stops us, shakes our hands and gives us a very sincere thank you.

Before we leave the ER, Ramon is transported to the cath lab. There, blood flow to his heart will be restored using the most advanced medical technology and procedures to be found anywhere in the world. I stop and look around the ER, take note of the dozens of people seeking medical care and the people there to give it to them. It looks like and sometimes is absolute chaos, but shining through all of that is the ingredient that makes me come back day after day, week after week and year after year. The people I work with make this the greatest job in the world. The firefighters, EMT's, housekeepers, nurses, technicians, secretaries, security and doctors all make me proud to be a part of this. Even Junior has a part.

"Still want to go to Engine 15?" I ask Mike as he puts the truck back together and I finish my report. We've spent the last three years working together, Mike and I. He's ten years younger, full of wit and sarcasm and a seemingly inexhaustible supply of energy. I see more of him than I do my family. During our previous shift,

Mike told me he plans on transferring from Rescue 1 to Engine 15. Life on the rescue beats you down if you let it, Mike has had enough. I have no idea how I manage - necessity, I guess.

"If all the calls were like this I might change my mind," he says as he hangs an IV set-up in its place over the stretcher. "That guy was having a heart attack!"

"He still is but it looks like he'll be all right."

We finish our tasks and get ready for more. I take the mic out of its cradle, hold it in my hand for a moment, and then press the key.

"*Rescue 1 in Service.*"

TWO

"I wonder what they're making for dinner," I ask Mike, as we cruise through the streets of Providence. The work force has abandoned the city in droves. They have returned to their suburban retreats leaving mostly the people who live here and us, for the time being. Later, the crowds will return to frequent the restaurants and maybe catch a show. As the night progresses, the nightclub scene takes off. Friday night belongs to the thousands of young people who inhabit the downtown clubs looking for fun.

"I saw Steve bring in some grocery bags. That can only mean one thing," he says.

"Mexican Chicken," we both say at once. "Again."

Most firefighters have at least one meal that they can put together; Steve's is Mexican Chicken, which he makes regularly. Normal people who have a hot meal prepared for them are thankful and appreciative. Not us. If Rachel Ray came to the station and made us a feast, somebody would complain.

"Do you think Venda is still open?" I ask Mike.

"Let's take a look," he responds and we head toward Federal Hill.

The truck phone rings.

"Rescue 1, Lieutenant Morse," I answer on the first ring. It is the Chief looking for people to work overtime. Easter Sunday is in two days, there are a lot of positions open. The fire department is required by contract to have ninety-two firefighters on duty at all times. If enough people don't volunteer for overtime, the Chiefs are forced to order us to work. When holidays approach, the maneuvering begins early as people jockey for position and try to get the day off. Substitutions, personal days and unused vacation time come in handy around the holidays. If you are not at work, you can't be ordered to stay goes the conventional wisdom.

"Mike," asks Chief Cochrane, "do you want to work tomorrow?"

He has a lot of calls to make and doesn't appreciate any nonsense or chitchat. Normally he will talk with "the guys" for hours. Most of our chief officers came up through the ranks, making Captain before being considered for advancement to the Chief's position. Those that make Chief are held in high regard by the people who once worked side by side with them. If you fight a fire or two with somebody bonds form that last a lifetime. Promotions to management usually can't change that.

"Yes sir."

"How about Leclaire?"

I hand the phone to Mike.

"Rescue 1, firefighter Leclair."

"Mike, can you work tomorrow?"

"Yes sir," he says. That seals our doom. We're stuck here for thirty-eight hours on a holiday weekend. The cab of the truck should be a barrel of laughs by Sunday morning. There is method to our madness. The Chiefs are reluctant to have anybody work more than three shifts in a row. If things go according to plan, we will be going home on Easter morning.

The Chief tells Mike our assignments. I'm going to Rescue 3 on Branch Avenue and Mike is going downtown to Rescue 4.

"I thought you weren't going to work," I say to him as we turn the corner onto Atwells Avenue.

"I need the money," Mike replies saying all that needs to be said. We travel up the Hill lost in our own thoughts. We will miss our families. The radio has gone silent for now. We find that Venda closed and head back to the station. I call Cheryl on the way.

"Hello."

"Hi babe, bad news, Venda is closed."

"I knew I should have gone myself. Why didn't you go yesterday?"

"I didn't have time; we've already been through this"

"You didn't have time to feed the dogs either. Or fix the sink. I told you it was leaking three days ago. It would only take a second if you would just do it. I may as well live by myself."

Here we go.

"If you're so smart, why don't you fix it yourself? Or call a plumber," I say.

"We can't afford a plumber. And you know I can't fix it."

"We should be able to afford a plumber, all I do is work, where is all the money."

"If you're so smart why don't you handle the bills?"

"Because I don't have time."

"Well I don't have time for this bullshit." She hangs up the phone. I only got beat by a second. I wish they had a sound effect of a phone slamming on cell phones. Pushing the off button hard loses it's impact.

"Trouble in paradise?" Mike asks.

"I thought you were leaving," I say.

"Couple of weeks."

"Great."

Two days ago I started my four-day work cycle. The morning I left home everything was great, life returned to normal after a four-day stretch with twenty-four hours not at work. Sleep deprivation plays tricks on your mind and puts a real strain on relationships. My family depends on me, but I'm seldom there, and when I am I'm either sleeping or wishing I was. The first half of my four-day shift is over, two nights and an overtime shift and I'll be back home. Easter Sunday is upon us, I'm supposed to get some homemade manicotti from the local Italian delicatessen. Not a big deal but it is my only contribution to the feast. Cheryl is certain I'll forget, and history is on her side. Will I forget? Never happen.

"Rescue 1 a still alarm."

1850 hrs. (6:50 p.m.)

"This will get your mind off of things," says Mike as we wait to hear what we have in store.

"Rescue 1, respond to Roger Williams Park in the vicinity of the Temple to Music for a two year old with blood and glass on his face. Unknown injuries."

"Rescue 1 responding."

We pick up 95 south from Atwells Avenue. The response time should be about five minutes. The sun has already set, but light is visible on the horizon casting an eerie glow. Pitch-blackness is hours away.

Roger Williams Park is full of activities for everybody. It is clean, well managed and nationally known and respected. There you will find one of the oldest zoos in the country, paddleboat rides, a carousel village, ponds, fields and woods. It is a safe place and a nice family destination. It is a good place to escape the rigors of city life and relax. Of course, there are exceptions. Now and then somebody gets murdered, or worse.

We leave the gritty neighborhood of South Providence behind, turn into the park and drive through the winding, hilly roads on the way to the Temple to Music. My parents' wedding pictures were taken there. Sometimes, after I've been up for a day or two, I can see them standing in the middle of the temple, just as they were in July of 1957. A lot has changed since then, I wish I could say for the better. I wonder when the seemingly endless decline of our society will finally hit bottom and start to climb, and if we will even notice when it does.

At the bottom of a rolling hill, on the edge of a spacious pond, sits the Temple. It is an open-air, marble structure of Greek-inspired architecture. Concerts are performed here as well as numerous other activities. My old friends, The Dropkick Murphys, perform here now and then. For decades this was the site of the state's finest Fourth of July fireworks display.

As we reach the crest of a hill overlooking the Temple it becomes apparent that fireworks of a different sort happened here. A two-year-old child being held in his mother's arms by the side of the road is screaming, his face a bloody mask. A car sits close by, all of the windows smashed. A young man - himself covered with blood - is talking to the police, who are doing a good job of calming him down. Mike pulls the rescue into the fray.

"What's going on here?" he asks as I walk toward the mother and child.

"We were driving through the park on our way home," the mother begins, while I look at her son's injuries, "two boys were getting beat up by about twenty people. My husband stopped the car and tried to help but they turned on him. They hit him with a baseball bat then smashed all of the windows in our car."

I've looked the boy over and can't find any injuries. Mike is checking the boy's father.

"Where did all of this blood come from?" I ask.

"His father was holding him after the crowd ran away. He was kissing him and he got his blood all over him."

"I don't see any injuries but let's go to the truck where I can clean him up and look a little closer."

I help the mother and child into the back of the rescue and moisten a towel with sterile water, gently dabbing the boy's face as he sobs. His mother, who has held herself together until now, finally lets loose a river of tears.

"I was so afraid, I thought they were going to kill us," she says between sobs.

"Your husband was very brave trying to help out like that. It's a good thing he only got beat up for his troubles, he could have been killed." I try to compliment her family while pointing out the danger they were in. I've finished checking the boy and find no injuries. He was sitting in the back seat sleeping in his car seat when the fracas began. Glass from the shattered windows landed on him but his mother was able to shake it off. The father is another story. I leave the two in the back of the rescue to check on the dad.

"Did you hear this one?" says Mike. "This guy's a hero. He beat off twenty armed attackers to save two kids he didn't even know."

The man's face is bruised and bloody. He has welts on his forearms where he must have fended off the bat attack. He is wiping his face with a towel Mike gave him while telling the police the story.

"We were just driving home through the park when I saw two kids, they couldn't have been more than fourteen, getting chased by a bunch of other kids, only the other kids were a little older. I thought they were fooling around, but they caught the little kids right next to my car and started beating them up bad. I couldn't just sit there so I got out, locked the car and tried to stop them. I stopped them all right. The boys ran away while one of the guys in the crowd attacked me with a baseball bat. Another one smashed all of the windows of my car. I think they ran off when they realized I had a baby in the car."

"Very chivalrous of them," I say.

"Can you describe the assailants?" The police officer asks.

"They were young, Hispanic guys. Probably Dominican," he says. I notice a Puerto Rican flag hanging from the destroyed car's rear view mirror.

"Do you want to press charges?"

"Do you think you'll catch them?" asks the man.

"Were going to try," says the officer. I can tell that he means it. Nobody wants to see good people getting attacked for trying to help somebody else. There is no reason for a nice family to be put through the torture these folks have endured. The police in Providence are a tough bunch, but their hearts are as big as the park we're in. Innocent people have been traumatized and that is unacceptable. Somehow, in some way the people responsible for this will be held accountable.

"They fucked with my family," says the man, "I want them to pay for that."

"Good man," says the cop. "We'll let you know when we have somebody to identify."

The police have their report, now they are going to get the bad guys.

"You should go to the hospital," I say. "You took a pretty bad beating."

"Are my son and wife okay?" he asks.

"Not a scratch," I tell him.

"That's good. I'll go to the hospital when I get them home and safe. I'll have my brother take me."

"Make sure you go. You might have a concussion."

"I'll be all right. I just want to go home," he says.

"That's what we all want." I tell him. He signs a refusal form for him and the boy. I shake his hand and wish him well as we go our separate ways.

THREE

"He's lucky to be alive," says Mike.

"I'll say. Imagine if that was you and Henry driving through the park. Would you have stopped to help those kids?"

"I really don't know."

"Neither do I. I guess you just respond to things when they come up. That guy probably never thought he would do what he did until he did it."

"He'd make a good firefighter," says Mike. "That's what we do; respond to things that come up. Other than that, we get paid to wait."

"What did you do before this?" I ask, surprised and embarrassed by the fact that I don't already know.

"Post Office. There is a reason so many people go crazy working there. It's pretty dull."

"I'll bet."

Darkness has descended on the city. The moon casts a phosphorescent glow, illuminating the ponds and fields with enough light to make their outlines visible as we pass. It is a beautiful night. The park is nearly deserted, with only the animals that inhabit the woods and zoo to keep us company as we drive through. A few cars pass us as they cut through from Broad Street to Elmwood Avenue, other than that the place is desolate. At times, working on the rescue gives you the same desolate feeling. The rest of the guys are back at the station watching TV, helping prepare the night's meal or doing whatever it is they do. They are together and the rescues are on the outside looking in. We usually miss the meal, which is when most of the bonding occurs. We never are able sit around shooting the shit or have time to watch a game or a movie. When we make it back to the station, we're tired and miserable or so far behind in the paperwork that it makes it hard to get into any kind of groove.

My fondest memories from the beginning of my career, when I was a firefighter working on an engine company, involve the conversations we would have. We found ways to solve world hunger, could run the Patriots, Red Sox or Bruins better than the bozos who called themselves coaches could, and knew the path toward world peace. The conversation was lively, informative and most important, hilarious. Most days the banter would begin over the coffee pot in the morning and go all day.

The rescues are in and out all day and never get into the flow of things. Entering into the ass end of a conversation makes you the ass of the conversation, I was told by an old firefighter, when I added my two cents to a conversation that I knew nothing about. It was good advice.

"Let's head back to quarters and see what's up," I say.

"Maybe we'll stay there for a while."

It is 1930 hrs, or 7:30 p.m. Just as we are walking up the stairs I hear a welcome announcement.

"All Hot!" blares from the stations PA system. We're just in time. It is Steve's turn to cook and - as expected - he has made his "Mexican Chicken." He puts some chicken breasts in a baking dish, covers them with salsa, tops that with cheddar cheese, then sprinkles some diced olives and scallions on top. With a little spicy rice on the side, we're ready for a fiesta. All that's missing are the Coronas.

"There are other things to eat than Mexican Chicken," says Jay.

"How did you get so fat if this is all you eat?" Captain Healy asks Steve, as he puts enough food on his plate to feed three men. He'll go back for seconds.

"People in fat houses shouldn't throw stones," responds Steve.

Arthur adds, "It is good Friday. Mexican fish would have been more appropriate."

"I forgot all about Good Friday!" says Steve. "I hope I don't go to hell."

"I've already been there," says the Captain as he takes a bite. "All they eat is Mexican Chicken. And all of the demons look just like you."

"That's not hell, that's heaven," says Steve. Suddenly, the blow lights come on and the P.A. system blares out the following.

"Attention Engines 10, 11, 13 Special Hazards, Ladders 5 and 2 and Battalion 2 a still box."

The members of Engine 13 drop everything and hit the poles. A still box means there is probably a fire. The P.A. system comes back with the rest.

"Engines 10, 11 and 13, Ladders 5 and 2, Special Hazards and Battalion 2, respond to 121 Moore Street for a reported structure fire."

"Let's head over there," I say.

"Why?" Mike asks.

"Because we're firemen and there's a fire," I say, sounding more annoyed than I intended.

"We used to be firemen, now we're rescue blows," Mike says.

"Once a fireman, always a fireman."

"Let's eat first," says Mike.

"If it's a code red get ready to roll," I say

A code red is our way of relaying the information to fire alarm and all responding companies that there is a working fire at the location and to proceed. Code yellow indicates a small fire or some other emergency that the first due companies will handle. Code blue means false alarm. We wait to hear the code while eating our chicken.

Fire alarm doesn't send a rescue until the fire is confirmed, or if there are multiple calls and they can tell the fire call is real. After fielding thousands of calls the dispatchers can sense which calls are legitimate from the ones that are not. I monitor the radio transmissions and wait to hear. I don't have to wait long as the radio transmits Engine 10's message:

"Engine 10 to fire alarm, we have a code yellow, food on the stove."

"Message received Engine 10; all other companies can go in service."

The person living on Moore Street probably left his dinner cooking and it caught fire. The apartment filled with smoke and somebody called 911. The fire department won't send just one truck when there is a report of a fire inside of a building. Better to err on the side of caution and have too many trucks and firefighters than not enough, especially when lives could be in jeopardy.

Mike and I finish our meals then cover the plates left on the table with foil. Mike cleans up the kitchen and I head to my office. The guys will be back to finish dinner and insult each other but I need some time to unwind. It's going to be a long night.

The Red Sox are on TV; I hope I get a chance to watch some of the game. For some weird reason, I liked the Red Sox more when they always broke the hearts of their fans. Something about getting what you wish for not always being a good thing comes to mind...

2209 hrs. (10:30 p.m.)

"Rescue 1 and Engine 9, Respond to 232 Power Street for a twelve year old male who fell down a flight of stairs."

It has been almost three hours since our last run. The break was welcome. I think the Sox won the game but I fell asleep while watching. Power Street runs next to the Brook Street fire station. The 9's should be on the scene quickly. Mike has the lights and sirens on as we speed toward the incident. Most of the time these calls are not life threatening, but injuries sustained on stairs can be critical. I want to get there quickly.

"Engine 9 to fire alarm, Inform Rescue 1 we have a twelve year old male, conscious and alert lying upside down at the bottom of a flight of stairs complaining of neck pain."

"Rescue 1, received."

The patient will need to be immobilized and transported to Hasbro. I don't have to tell Mike anything, he knows what to do. When we arrive on scene I go inside while Mike and Mark, one of the firefighters from Engine 9, prepare the backboard, collar and necessary straps needed for extrication. I walk up ten cement steps, through an ornate doorway and into the home. The patient is lying at the bottom of a wooden staircase, upside down. The smells of past centuries linger in the hall, musty and mysterious. A plaque marking this as a historic home is proudly displayed on the exterior. The name of the builder or owner, most likely one in the same, is engraved on the plaque along with the year the house was built, 1838. I wonder if any ghosts are watching.

The patient is lying on his back looking up at the ceiling. His mother sits a few steps above the boy. She tells me what happened.

"He was running down the stairs like he always does only this time he tripped and fell down."

"Did you see him fall?" I ask.

"Of course, I was right behind him."

"Did he slide down the steps or roll over and over, like tumbling?"

"Oh, he tumbled all right. He fell forward then flipped over and landed right there. He hasn't moved."

How many steps did he fall down?"

"About eight."

"Did he lose consciousness?"

"No, but he won't move."

"Won't, or can't?"

"Won't."

"What is his name?"

"David."

I crouch next to David to do an initial assessment.

"Can you move?" I ask.

"I don't know, I haven't tried," he responds.

"How will you know if you don't try?" I ask.

"I don't want to slip into a coma," he says, deathly serious.

"Are you feeling any pain?" I ask while looking him over to see if there are any gross deformities. There are not.

"No, but I might be slipping into a coma."

"What makes you think that?"

"Because people always go into comas."

"No they don't," I say.

"Yes they do," he responds.

"Comas aren't so bad."

"How do you know?"

"I don't for sure, but they don't look all that bad."

Mark and Mike have retrieved the backboard and collar from the truck, place the board next to him and apply the cervical collar. Starting from his head, I work my way up his entire body, asking if he feels pain and feeling for any sign of trauma. It will be impossible to extricate him without moving him a little. He has to lie flat on the backboard. I hold David's head, keeping the neck aligned with the rest of him as Mike holds his hips and Mark gets the legs. Pat gets the long board in place and prepares to place it under the patient.

"On three roll him onto his side," I direct the guys. "One, two, three." When I say three, we all move together, placing David on his side while Pat slides the board underneath.

"On three roll him back. One, two, three." As one we put him onto the board. Straps are used to hold him in place. In about a minute we have him immobilized and are ready to carry him to the truck.

"Am I in a coma?" David asks.

"Nope, you're just tied up like a mummy. A coma might be better," I tell him, as we carry him from the house and into the rescue. Once there, I evaluate his vital signs and do a basic neurological assessment.

"Squeeze my hands," I tell him, as I put my hands into his.

He squeezes hard enough to crack my finger bones, both sides equally.

"Push your foot forward like you're stepping on the gas," I say, placing my hand on the bottom of his foot.

"I'm twelve, I don't drive," he says.

"And you've never driven a bumper car or a go cart?" I ask.

"I might crash and go into a coma."

"Just push, will you!" He does. I put my hands on top of his feet and ask him to pull back. He does that too. He has pulses in both of his feet. We're ready to transport him to Hasbro. From the look of things he was lucky. There doesn't appear to be any damage to his body, and his fear of slipping into a coma is probably temporary.

David's mother comes with us as we transport. She doesn't seem too concerned.

"Have you been through this before?" I ask her.

"How could you tell?" she responds.

"Intuition I guess. You're not acting like this is the first time he has been in this position."

"He's never ended up in a rescue, but he's constantly falling and worrying he's paralyzed or slipping into a coma."

"I'm sure he'll be fine," I say to both of them.

"I'm sure too," says his mom.

"You're not the ones slipping into a coma," says David, his eyes fluttering, the weight of an uncertain future lingering over him. His mom and I can't help ourselves and laugh out loud.

Heidi is at the triage desk at Hasbro. I tell her the story, emphasizing David's fear of slipping into a coma. I don't know if he is being dramatic or is really afraid. I get the feeling he is toying with us a little, having some fun and getting attention. I don't mind a bit, I'm happy he wasn't injured more severely. The speed at which life changes is incredible. Nobody ever sees it coming.

We transfer David from our stretcher to the one waiting for us at the hospital. Heidi has just finished the latest installment in Stephen King's series, *The Gunslinger*. One of the best things about reading a good book is finding somebody else that has shared the experience.

FOUR

While driving back to quarters, Mike's body goes into convulsions. He looks at me with crossed eyes and says, "I think I'm going into a coma!"

"Cut that out and drive, you idiot," I say.

"I'm not an idiot, I'm a human being," he says while holding his left arm up to his nose, simulating an elephant's trunk. "I am not an animal!"

"You're the elephant man!" I say. It's going to be a long night. I take my phone from my top pocket and call home.

"Hello."

As the years progress in any relationship, simple words begin to have multiple meanings. The tones and inflections used when speaking a word such as "hello" give the word power it really doesn't deserve. This particular "hello" shouts, "prepare to die." I decide to retreat and take a defensive position.

"Hi babe, how is your night?"

"Easter is the day after tomorrow, the house is a mess, I haven't done any shopping and you're asking how my night is."

"Have the kids help."

"Brittany is out, Danielle has her own life and you're at work. That leaves me to do everything. As usual."

"We appreciate it." I say, knowing it is much too late for compliments but unable to stop.

"Bullshit. If you appreciated it so much you wouldn't have forgotten the manicotti."

She's hitting a nerve. Time to break cover.

"What, do you think this is easy? I've been busting my balls over here and all you do is complain."

"I'd rather do your job than stay in this house."

"Be careful what you wish for."

"I've got too much to do. I'm not wasting time talking nonsense with you."

"Fine."

"Fine."

This battle has ended with no victor. I have a feeling the war is not over. I hang up first, then pick up the radio mic and go in service. It is still in my hand when it talks back.

2320 hrs. (11:20 p.m.)

"Rescue 1, respond to 385 Mawney Street for a man hearing voices."

"Rescue 1 responding."

"I'm hearing voices too. My wife's. And it ain't pretty." I mumble to myself.

"You love it," says Mike. I can't even have a conversation with myself in this stupid truck.

"No I don't. I hate when she gets like this."

"They all get crazy around the holidays, you're not special."

"My wife is worse," I say.

"I'm telling you, they're all nuts."

"Women."

"Women."

There is a patient who is hearing voices waiting for us at Mawney Street. I have no idea if those voices are telling him to kill the rescue guys when they get there.

"Rescue 1 to fire alarm, are the police responding?"
"They have been notified."
"Message received."

People suffering with mental illness such as bi-polar disorder and schizophrenia are able to lead productive lives. While medication has proven effective in treating these disorders, often, after the medication has been able to work, the patient takes himself off of the meds and ends up an emotional ruin. The patient's family or caseworkers need to get them to a medical facility but they are extremely uncooperative. The families call 911 for transport. I don't know what the public expects from us when we get there, I have no training in restraining uncooperative patients, and only a basic understanding of mental illness. The patients are volatile. Police are called, and if the patient is completely out of their mind, will help us restrain the patient for their own safety and come with us in the back of the truck during transport. If the patient is stable, we take them in and hope things don't get out of control. If I were to restrain every emotional patient that I felt had the potential to get violent, half of the people I transport would be tied down.

We pull the rescue in front of an old, decrepit apartment building. I have been to this address numerous times for calls ranging from murders to drunks. Outside, a man and woman are waiting. The woman hails us as if we were a cab. The truck has barely stopped as the two reach for the rear door handle to let themselves in. The truck stops and I get out and confront them.

"What are you doing?" I ask, moving the man's hand off of the door handle.

"I called for a rescue, what do you mean, what am I doing," he says. His eyes are wild, giving him a menacing appearance.

"What do you think this is, a cab company?" I ask.

"You've got to take him to Butler," the woman with him demands.

Butler Hospital is a psychiatric hospital located on the Seekonk River in the city's East Side. They don't accept patients from rescues, only walk-ins and physician referrals.

"We can't take him to Butler," I say. "If he needs to be seen, we can take him to Rhode Island Hospital for a psych evaluation and they will take him to Butler."

"I'm not going to Rhode Island, they don't do nothing," he says.

"You better go, you been hearin' voices again. I ain't goin' through that bullshit ever." She turns to me and demands I take him to Butler. Mike has joined me outside the truck and asks some questions.

"What is the problem?" The two people ignore me and talk to Mike. Lunatics always seek each other out.

"He hasn't been taking his meds for a week," the woman explains, "then this morning he told me the voices are telling him things."

"What kind of things?" Mike asks.

"They're telling me to hurt myself and other stuff too," he says. "I need to go to Butler."

"Do you have a plan?" I ask. One of the criteria for emergency medical treatment for psychiatric emergencies is whether or not the patient has a plan to carry out any suicidal thoughts.

"Yeah, I got a plan," he says. "I plan on going to Butler."

Why I get myself into these things is beyond me.

"Get in the truck." I say, and they do.

"And don't sit in that seat," I say, while pointing to my seat. They all want to sit in my seat, it drives me crazy.

Once inside and sitting on the bench seat the man appears to have relaxed. Mike starts to asses his vital signs and I attempt to explain things to him again.

"We're going to take you to Rhode Island where they will give you an evaluation then transfer you over to Butler. That is the best we can do. Now that you have told me you are suicidal and have a plan to carry out those wishes, we have to make sure you get some help. I know it isn't exactly what you wanted, but it's the best we can do."

"Well why didn't you say so?" the woman asks as she prepares to leave the back of the truck.

"Where are you going?" I ask.

"I'm going to meet him there later," she says and walks away.

The trip to Rhode Island takes about three minutes. Again, I ask myself if anybody in this city is able to take care of themselves.

My patient is a thirty-year-old male with a history of bi-polar disorder and depression. He is supposed to be taking numerous psych medications, but feels he is cured and no longer needs them. As soon as the medication wears off, the symptoms return. It looks as though he is ready to go into the manic part of his disease. Anything can happen at this point. If the trip to the hospital were any longer I would wait for the police, but I am reasonably certain I can get him there without incident. In the event that he attacks me, Mike is ready to speed the truck up rapidly. For the patient to get from the bench seat over to where I am seated, he has to stand up. As soon as Mike steps on the gas, he'll go flying. At that point, I can either abandon ship and leave the guy alone in the truck or wrap him up in a sheet and ride the rest of the way while sitting on top of him. It is not a fool-proof method, but it has worked in the past. My preferred method is to keep the patient calm by talking. People love it when somebody listens, and our transport time is so short he won't have time to get sick of me.

I am relieved when I feel the familiar bumps in the road and know we are backing into the rescue bay. Mike has alerted ER security to stand by; we have a possibly combative patient. Two guards, Amir and Steve are waiting. The hospital couldn't have picked better guys; both can handle themselves without a problem, but more importantly they know how to talk the patients into staying in line. This patient may be beyond reason, so I alert them of that possibility before talking to the triage nurse. Gary is back; I'm batting a thousand. He takes the report, and then moves the patient into the observation area without incident. Steve and Amir stand by holding four point restraints. It looks as though they won't be needed, but it is better to be safe. People have gone berserk here with no warning. A doctor will do an evaluation soon and the patient will probably be transferred to Butler. In the meantime, the hospital is responsible for his well being. I'm just glad we got him here without incident. I can't help but think of an incident on Broad Street that happened to a social worker late last year. He was on a routine visit to a psych patient's home. The social worker, a guy in his forties with a wife and two kids, finished his evaluation and felt that his patient wasn't doing well and should be seen at a hospital. While they waited for a rescue to arrive, the patient took a screwdriver and stabbed the social worker in the neck, killing him instantly.

FIVE

It's Friday night at midnight and all five of Providence's rescues are busy at Rhode Island Hospital. Well over half of our runs tonight will be alcohol related. Rescue 2 has brought an intoxicated male in from Cranston Street. He was found lying in a doorway, unconscious. Rescue 3 has a drunken Providence College student with them. I prefer the seasoned drunks like Darryl and Leroy; they never puke in the back of the truck. College kids either want to kill you when they are drunk, or they throw up without warning, usually all over the equipment. We always place an emesis basin in quick reach on weekend nights. Rescue 4 has brought in an assault victim from one of the downtown clubs and Rescue 5 has a RISD student who may have overdosed.

The radio chatter continues, sending out of town rescues into the city. While the revelers continue to party, real medical emergencies occur. An East Providence rescue heads to Wickenden Street for an elderly woman with chest pains, a Johnston rescue responds to Killingly Street for a four-year-old having a seizure and Cranston Rescue 2 is on the way to Broad Street. From the sound of our dispatch, they're going to get Darryl. Again.

The triage area is out of control. People with assorted injuries occupy twenty of the stretchers that fill the room, some on spine boards with cervical collars around their necks, others just lying on the stretchers. A few elderly people are nestled in among the drunks and injured. Some seem amused by the circus around them, others not so much. There, everybody waits until a spot in the treatment area opens up. The seriously injured are in trauma alley.

The night is young and already the hospital is overburdened. Tanya is working with Gary and they are doing their best to keep up with the steady flow of patients coming through the doors. They not only have to contend with the rescues, but are responsible for walk-ins as well.

Outside, the cool, evening air offers a welcome change from the stifling atmosphere of the ER. I join the rest of the rescue crews who have gathered around the trucks. Theresa and Tim from Rescue 5 sit on the rear bumper of their truck, Zack and Mike from Rescue 4, Isaac and Chris from Rescue 2 and Heidi and Al from Rescue 3 are all here, standing around swapping stories and having some laughs, waiting for the next call. This is our bonding time. The firefighters are back in the stations, all of the rescues are here. It is a nice diversion from a night full of stress and aggravation to get together and vent. Most of the talk is about the nitwits we have been taking to the hospital, or how many runs we've had. It is an important and vital part of a busy night to get together and see that we are not alone. The ten people working the rescues will do seventy-five percent of the fire department's work tonight.

Two by two our numbers dwindle. First Heidi and Al go to an accident on Branch Avenue. Tim and Theresa are next; another assault at a downtown club. Isaac and Chris get sent to Poccasset Avenue for an asthma attack and Zack and Mike head downtown for some hot wieners at Haven Brothers. Mike and I decline their invitation and head back to quarters, hoping to get some rest before things get busy again.

I consider calling Cheryl to say goodnight but decide to let it rest. Tomorrow we'll try again.

0136 hrs. (1:36 a.m.)

"Rescue 1; respond to 1016 Babcock Street for a domestic disturbance, stage for police."

I put the book I was reading down and head for the truck. Domestic disturbances can be horrendous. Not only do we have to deal with injured people, but the people doing the injuring as well. Sometimes the assailants remain on the scene and cause problems for us. The police are called first to quiet things down, and then call us in if we are needed.

"What's on the scanner?" Mike asks as we drive toward the incident.

"Let's find out," I say and flip the switch on the police scanner we have mounted under ours. Fire and police frequencies are different, we can't communicate with them directly, nor they with us, but we are able to monitor their transmissions. There is no news from Babcock, just cruisers being sent throughout the city for different reasons. The police work differently than the fire department. The volume of calls they receive make it impossible for them to respond instantly to calls for help. They use a priority basis; this domestic must not be high priority. The fire department responds instantly to the calls we receive with all available resources needed for the incident. If we are not able to muster an adequate response, mutual aid will be called from surrounding communities until all resources have been depleted. That has never happened.

We keep the lights and siren off during our response, and then stage a safe distance from the house on Babcock. I hope nobody there needs immediate medical assistance. I have no intention of going into a domestic dispute unarmed. The emotions are too high and alcohol and drugs are probably a part of the problem making matters worse. It's funny what pops in your mind while waiting.

The three little girls sat on a couch in their living room, holding hands. They were afraid. I gave them a smile as I walked through the room and into the kitchen. They didn't smile back. A woman, possibly their mother lay on the floor, a hole in the middle of her forehead. A gun was on the floor a few feet away from her. Lt. Segee stood off to the side, shook his head when he saw me approach the patient.

"Too late," he said.

A man in handcuffs stood off to the side, catatonic, or pretending to be. There was no need to feel for a pulse or run a strip, the woman was obviously dead. No sense contaminating the crime scene any more than it already was. One of the police officers asked me to "look at" their prisoner. He had gone to a place deep inside himself and wasn't coming back anytime soon. We stepped around the remains of what should have been the man's ex-wife, now a murder victim.

We walked him past the three little girls, crying now, the safe world they knew gone forever.

From the police scanner, I hear a car being dispatched to the scene. A few minutes later, one car appears in the distance with lights flashing but no siren. Another cruiser passes our position and turns down Babcock Street. Rescue 1 stays put until the police sort things out. A few minutes later the officer on scene reports there are no injuries and the rescue won't be needed. I hope this is a happy ending for the people involved, not just a stay of execution.

The bars just closed, letting hordes of drunken fools loose into the city. I don't think we'll be in quarters for long.

SIX

"Rescue 1, Respond to 329 Parkis Street for a four-year-old, vomiting."

0334 hrs. (3:34 a.m.)

"Rescue 1 responding."

I can't believe that it is already 3:30. The bar crowd has departed the city without calling us. I had turned my radio off and slept for an hour or so and missed hearing if any of the other rescues responded to calls. I'm sure that they did.

Years ago I partied at the same downtown clubs that are popular today, but I have no recollection of any fire department responses during my visits. I do recall a few incidents with the police, but those are stories best told another day.

My generation was more self-reliant than the kids who go to the clubs today. We took care of each other. Kids today would rather call 911 and leave their drunken or injured friends in the back of a rescue with strangers than take responsibility for them.

Some of the clubs in Providence are not friendly places. Fights are rampant. Ecstasy calmed things down for a while, but that craze has died down, with cocaine becoming more popular. I miss the Ecstasy. The kids all loved each other and were too wasted to fight or cause much trouble. Now, every night somebody gets a beating. Rescues are called and often find heavily intoxicated people with bloody noses, or swollen eyes and bumps on their heads. It is state protocol for all emergency personnel to transport patients with head injuries to the emergency room only after applying a cervical collar and placing them on a backboard. This setup presents numerous problems. For one, the patients are inexperienced drinkers. Traveling in the back of a truck, lying backwards with their neck immobilized is a sure recipe for a disaster. The patients sometimes have to throw up, but are lying on their back and can't turn their head. We are supposed to keep them immobilized during transport, but that becomes impossible. Allowing somebody to drown in his or her vomit is counter-productive. The patients are usually very uncooperative. People with head injuries can be difficult to begin with; add alcohol to the mix and they are impossible. Often we need a fire company to assist us on scene. The firefighters hold the patients onto the stretcher and provide necessary manpower in restraining people who become combative. I am glad we managed to escape all of this tonight.

We have pulled the truck in front of what once was a respectable apartment building but is now a crack house. The four-year-old who is vomiting is inside this shithole, somewhere. Mike and I walk gingerly up five rotted wooden steps onto a sagging porch. The front door is more secure than a bank vault. Six doorbells are on the right side of the entryway; I don't know which apartment the patient is in, so I push all six. After a minute a voice comes over an intercom.

"Who's there?" the voice asks

"Providence Rescue," I respond.

"How do I know you're the rescue?"

"Are you near a front window?" I ask.

"Yeah," comes the tinny reply.

"Look outside."

"Hold on."

"Do you see the rescue and all the flashing lights?"

"Yeah."

"Then who the hell do you think we are?" I ask. A buzzing sound comes from the front door allowing me to push it open.

"Rescue 1 on scene," I tell fire alarm. If we disappear I want somebody to know where we were last seen.

The hallway is dark. Tenants steal the light bulbs from the fixtures as soon as the landlord replaces them. Mike lights the way with a tiny penlight. The smell of smoke, body odor and stale booze permeates the narrow passageway.

"Rescue 1 to fire alarm, do you have an apartment number?"

"Roger Rescue 1, Apartment 102."

"Received."

Mike flashes his beam onto barricaded doors as we walk past - 102 is at the end of the hall, past a stairway that leads to upstairs apartments. The building is zoned for six units, but I'd bet the rescue there are at least ten apartments here. The population of Providence is exploding, but affordable housing is not keeping pace. Illegal apartments have become a huge problem. I knock on the door of apartment 102, hear some shuffling, then the door opens, letting a plume of marijuana smoke into the hall. A young man wearing nothing but piss-stained jockeys leads me into a two-room apartment over to a bare mattress lying in the corner of the "living" room. Dirty dishes lie about; spent cigarette butts sharing the dish surface with mold covered food. The walls are crawling with cockroaches and an army of flies is feeding on cat, dog and human feces that litter the floor. On the bed is a beautiful four-year-old girl, sweating and pale, with a vomit filled bucket perched next to her. The pail looks ready to spill onto her and the mattress and may already have.

"What is going on here?" I ask the man who answered the door.

"I don't know. Her mother dropped her off at eight. She's been crying and puking non stop since."

"She's sick," I say, while moving the bucket of vomit away from her. "Mike, get a clean blanket from the truck." He looks glad to get out of the stinking place.

"What is her name?"

"Cassandra. You gonna fix her?" Underwear Man asks.

"I'm taking her to Hasbro. She needs to be seen by a doctor," I say.

"Don't you got no medicine or nothin to give her?" he asks. Mike has returned with the blanket and wastes no time wrapping the little girl in it. She looks at him with glazed eyes and miraculously smiles.

"Take her to the truck, I'll be right out," I say to Mike. He carries her out. The girl doesn't look back. I radio fire alarm and request the police to meet us at Hasbro. This is a blatant case of child neglect. There isn't much I can do, only report my findings to the proper authorities

"What is the matter with you, letting a little kid live like this?" I ask

"Like what?" he asks.

"Like an animal."

"Fuck you man, you can't talk to me like that."

"Let's go."

"Where are we going?"

"To Hasbro."

"Bullshit, we're staying here."

"Look buddy, your daughter can't stay here. She's sick and needs medical attention. I can't leave her here, and you don't have a choice. Now let's go."

Reluctantly, he gets dressed and follows me to the rescue. Mike has Cassandra wrapped up tight and sleeping on the stretcher.

"She's got a temperature of 104, BP 140 over 78 and a pulse of 120," he says.

"Have you given her any medicine?" I ask Underwear Man.

"I can't afford no medicine."

"But can afford pot and cigarettes."

"That's none of your business."

"Yes it is."

I'm done talking to this piece of shit. When I get to Hasbro, I'll inform them of the deplorable living conditions and they will alert the State Department of Children, Youth and Families. Cassandra will probably be placed in a foster home until a caseworker can be assigned to them. The police will file a report. I don't know what will happen to the father, but if I had my way he would be locked up for good.

"Do you believe this shit?" says Mike as we leave Hasbro and head toward the station.

"We're here, away from our families trying to make a living and that asshole is home with his kid, who knows where the mother is. That girl was burning up and he sits around smoking reefer like there isn't a care in the world. Fuck him and fuck the mother and fuck everybody who lives in that piece of shit hellhole. They should be locked up. For good. I wish I could take that kid home."

I let Mike vent. There really isn't anything I can add to his diatribe - I feel the same way. I worry when the job gets to him. Things are pretty bad to get through his thick skin. His family means the world to him; it is unfathomable when he sees other people who just take it all for granted. I feel the same way.

It is impossible to forget the things we see. At some level, the sights, smells, sounds and emotions are with us for the rest of our lives. At any time, anywhere something could trigger a flashback, and what was a pleasant night at home, relaxing day at the beach or a nice dinner with friends suddenly loses its luster. It's taken me years to realize why.

SEVEN

The city is quiet. A few cars are with us on the road and I can hear the hum of tractor-trailers in the distance as they cruise down 95. Some thin clouds obscure the moon and stars, but for the most part they are visible, casting a serene glow over the sleeping city.

Alas, not all of the city sleeps. Half a mile from Hasbro I see Frankenstein's Monster stumbling down Eddy Street.

0400hrs. (4:00 a.m.)

"Rescue 1 to fire alarm, hold us out of service, Armand is loose."
"Roger Rescue 1, at 0400."

I don't need to give the dispatchers any more information; they are familiar with Armand. He is another of the many homeless alcoholics who roam the city. It is unusual to see him at this late hour; I want to make sure he is all right. Mike pulls the rescue close to him and I unroll the window. Armand keeps on trucking. The toes of both of his feet were amputated last winter because of frostbite, as well as all of his fingers on his right hand. Three of his left fingers are gone as well, amputated from the second knuckle.

When sober, his movements are a little unusual; when intoxicated he is the spitting image of the famous monster.

"Hey Armand, where are you going?" I ask. He raises his right hand and waves us off.

"Don't go making fists at me," I say. Without fingers, his wave looks like a fist shaking.

Suddenly, he stops walking, falls to his knees then rolls onto the sidewalk. It appears he has had enough.

"Let's get him," says Mike.

We leave the cab, glove up and go get him. Mike takes the feet and I get the shoulders.

"On three. One, two, three." I say and we lift him off the pavement.

We carry him to the back of the truck and lay him on the floor. No sense wasting clean linens, he is filthy. I get in back with him and Mike drives us to Rhode Island Hospital, which is right next to Hasbro.

"What's up, Armand?" I ask.

"The shelter's closed," he slurs. "Take me to the hospital."

"We're already there," I tell him. Mike has backed the truck into the rescue bay and is retrieving a stretcher from the triage area.

Armand is my favorite drunk. He is an educated man, or so he tells me, who lost his wife years ago and has been drinking himself to death since. When they are not lost or broken, he wears a pair of wire-rimmed glasses, giving him a distinguished look. At one time he was a welder and held a job at Electric Boat working on submarines. Rumor has it that he lives on a trust fund and has a wealthy sister who handles his money. It is only a matter of time that we will find him dead. He has lost the will to live. As he says, "I don't give a fuck."

Something must have snapped for him to become so despondent. He treats his body with reckless disregard. The frostbite from last year resulted in his fingers and toes being amputated. His disfigurement is obvious. The damage done to his soul is much more devastating and will be the cause of his early demise.

Mike opens the rear doors of the rescue. I keep Armand's head safe and Mike grabs him by the belt and drags him onto the hospital stretcher. We wheel him in. Tanya takes one look at our cargo and says, "We just let him go."

"I can't leave him lying on the sidewalk," I say.

"What's wrong with him?" she asks.

"He collapsed."

"Bring him in," she says with an exasperated sigh.

There is no reason for Armand to be here other than he has nowhere else to go. I don't know why the hospital released him in the middle of a cold spring night. I wish there was a better way to care for the indigents who plague the health care system, the present method is sorely lacking. Incarceration may be the safest for the patient and most cost effective for society.

It's late, I'm tired and I have had enough for one night. Mike drives back to the station. I turn the volume on the radio up when the DJ plays Lynard Skynard's brilliant Sweet Home Alabama.

EIGHT

I have had only an hour's sleep since yesterday, yet find it impossible to relax. Tonight's events, while disturbing, shouldn't be enough to deny me some needed rest, but that rest remains elusive. It's five a.m. and I have twenty-six hours to go, just being in the station causes insomnia. In two hours I'll make the journey to Branch Avenue to take over the reins of Rescue 3. Overtime is great, but it takes its toll on the mind and body. At this stage of a long shift, I have a tendency to fall into depression. The end is nowhere in sight and the calls are relentless. In the quiet confines of my office, I see the first traces of light filter through the blinds covering my window. I know I need the rest but my mind refuses to relent, instead choosing to replay the events of the week. The drunks, overdoses, medical emergencies and trauma, in addition to the loneliness and despair evident in so many that we come in contact with refuse to sit quietly in my mind. I know that my presence in their lives is miniscule and more than likely forgotten as soon as I leave the people I am called to help, but I hope that I have been able to alleviate their misery to some degree. The kids bother me the most. They have no idea of what life could be, only believe what they are shown by their elders. As their lives progress and experience grows, I can only hope that they can see some good in the world and aspire toward it. For now, I must witness their existence in the hellholes they call home and hope for a miracle.

My wife is home, sleeping by herself in our bed, the effects of her disease contributing to her loneliness as it continues on its destructive path. As her mobility decreases her world gets smaller and her dependency on me grows, only I'm not there, leaving her alone to deal with something nobody should have to face. Multiple Sclerosis is a bitch.

0623 hrs. (6:23 a.m.)
"Rescue1, Respond to the intersection of Broad and West Friendship for a woman with a head injury."

The last thing I remember is feeling sorry for myself. I must have fallen asleep while wallowing in self-pity. I'm glad I got that out of the way. The blow lights have come on, filling the station with fluorescent light. They stay on for one minute, then automatically shut off as I make my way down the stairs and toward the rescue. The morning is upon us and gives enough light for me to find my way, although I could find it in my sleep - and often do. Mike is already in the truck and has the motor running. He looks refreshed, as though he has had a full nights sleep. I look at him and shake my head.

"Sleep well?" he asks.

"Like a baby," I lie.

The door opens and we are again on our way toward Broad Street. This time we are headed to an area where prostitution and drug dealing are done openly on the street. I try to remain objective as we make our way to the patient. She may be an innocent victim of crime, or have just had an accident. The streets are mostly deserted; everybody must have found their way home, everyone except for the person who called for help. She waits on the corner of Broad and West Friendship, her clothes torn and hanging from her body and blood rushing down her face. She stands in the street calmly as we stop the rescue near her, get out and walk toward her.

"What happened?" I ask.

Her reply is so softly spoken that I cannot understand her. Mike has brought a sheet with him and wraps it around her like a cape. The woman clutches it around her neck. Only then do I notice the tears streaming down her face. We help her into the truck and close the door. Mike examines her head wound, controls the bleeding and reports his findings.

"She has a two inch laceration to the top of her head, on top of a large bump. It looks like somebody clubbed her over the head."

"Do you remember what happened?" I ask her.

"I was raped," comes her reply.

"Rescue 1 to fire alarm, have the police respond to this location."

"Received, Rescue 1. Nature for the police?"

"Possible sexual assault."

"Message received."

"Do you know who did it?" I ask.

"No."

"We have to take you to the hospital. Did you lose consciousness when you got hit in the head?" I ask

"I think so."

I get a cervical collar and gently put it around her neck. Mike has retrieved a long board from the side compartment and lays it on the stretcher while the patient stands up. She sits on the board in the middle then lies back, me cradling her head and back as she eases to a flat position. The tears continue to flow.

A series of loud knocks comes from the rear of the truck. Mike opens the door and a man tries to get in.

"Who are you?" Mike asks.

"What happened to you?" the man asks our patient in an impatient way, ignoring Mike.

"Are you family?" Mike asks.

"Yeah I'm her daddy, now shut up and let me talk to my girl," he says. Mike closes the door. Hard. The man is done knocking and leaves the scene right before the police arrive. The side door opens and a rookie officer sticks his head into the rescue, takes a look at the patient and shakes his head.

"Do you know her?" I ask.

"Everybody knows her. What happened sweetheart, deal gone bad?" He carries himself as though he has forty years on the streets and has seen it all. His smug grin transforms his good looks into a sneer that gives him the appearance of a punk. If I were to guess, he comes from the suburbs, played quarterback on his high school football team and wouldn't know a thing about hard knocks if they were trampling down his door.

"Where are you taking her?"

"Rhode Island ER."

"I'll meet you there." The cop leaves but his attitude lingers.

"What is your name?" I ask.

"Destiny."

"Mike is going to take your vital signs and we'll get going. The people at the hospital will take care of you."

"Nobody takes care of me," she says. "Nobody gives a shit"

"You're wrong. Right here, right now, you are the only person that matters to me. After I drop you off at the hospital that will change, but for now your best interests are all that I care about. I don't give a shit about the cops or the pimps or the asshole that beat you. I don't know who you are or what happened in your life for you to end up out here and it's none of my business, but I do care about is what is happening now and how I can make it better. Now shut up and let Mike take your vitals."

I don't know whether or not she believes me, but she seems to have settled down. Mike finishes with her, gives me her signs and goes to the front to drive. Life is not easy. Without a few breaks, good parenting and education, it is easy to fall into the many traps life has waiting to snare people without the skills to avoid them. Destiny would rather be anywhere than here, addicted to heroin and selling herself on the streets. If more people begin to give a shit and stop being so judgmental, her future may brighten. The odds are against her. There are a lot of kids in this city teetering on the edge of respectability or despair. A push in either direction will land them on their feet - or on their ass.

Heroin is cheap and readily available in Providence. It can be snorted through the nose or injected into a vein. The euphoria only lasts for a little while and then it's back to reality, a reality that most junkies prefer to forget. The drug takes a person's dignity, confidence and productiveness and leaves a shell where a human being once was. The spirit can and sometimes does reappear, but it is rare and sometimes fleeting. Once a junkie, always a junkie is the common perception, harsh, but unfortunately true. Some addicts manage to leave it all behind and go on to lead normal lives, most crash.

It is a selfish, lonely world the addicts live in. I've seen people left for dead in cars, apartments, fields; anywhere people gather to do their drugs. Every man for himself when somebody overdoses.

Keeping a job while under the influence of heroin is next to impossible. The users are forced to go underground. Selling the drug to other addicts is one way to get by, selling your body another.

Our prisons are full. A large number of inmates are incarcerated because of drug related crimes. The numbers don't tell the entire story. The robberies, B&E's, muggings, prostitution and scams are in large part devices used to obtain drugs. Legalizing the drugs would lead to more problems. Imagine if every drug dealer on the streets suddenly lost his income. The only way they know how to get by is by doing something illegal. Flipping burgers is unacceptable for this segment of the population; they see themselves as a cut above the common man. Maybe if they traded their fancy Cadillac Escalades and Lincoln navigators for a Ford pick-up truck or Chevy Blazer, and decided to cut lawns, clean offices of find some other line of honest work, the experience and work ethic would grow and they would become respectable members of society. Problem is, nobody wants to start at the bottom and work their way up. The riches available by leading a life of crime are too tempting to those afraid of work. Take the easy route of dealing drugs away and watch our other crime rates soar.

I should be going home; instead I'm looking at twenty-four more hours in Providence.

PART II

SATURDAY

NINE

Destiny is at the hospital in good hands. My guess is she will be back on the streets tomorrow. What connection we had will be forgotten as soon as somebody else comes into her life. I can only hope that what little kindness I showed her stays with her for a little while, at least.

Mike will be working at Rescue 4 and I am headed to Rescue 3. The ride between stations gives me an opportunity to unwind. There is no chance of getting a run now, I've left my radio with Tim and have some time to myself. The ride only lasts for about fifteen minutes, but those fifteen minutes of peace are vital components of a thirty-eight hour shift. With twenty-four hours to go survival becomes an hourly quest. The mundane runs wear you down until a true emergency tests your resolve. So far, I've been able to rise to the occasion when called upon and will leave the rescue division if I find I cannot.

The ride goes quickly, traffic on a Saturday morning light. The garage door is open, waiting for the day shift to enter. I pull in and turn the key off end enjoy a few moments of serenity in the basement of the Branch Avenue fire station. I am hoping for a quiet morning. As I reach into my back seat to get my bag, the speaker in the basement begins to bark. I can barely hear what is being said, but I'm sure it is another rescue run. My plan for a cup of coffee and some conversation with my friends from D group will have to wait.

0738 hrs. (7:38 a.m.)

"Rescue 3; respond to the Dexter Manor for an unknown medical problem."
Rick, the officer of Rescue 3, C group is more than ready to head home. He waits for me on the bottom landing of the stairs and hands me the portable as I pass.
"See you at five," he says, and then heads out the door. Usually talkative the night shift must have taken its toll on his spirit. My own spirit is quickly evaporating. I wish I hadn't said yes to the overtime. If it had been offered this morning, I would have said no. They always call as soon as I get to work when I still have some fuel in the tank. Right now I'm running on empty.
"What's up, Big Head," says Al, my partner for the day.
"Not much, Shrek," I reply. They could call us heavy rescue. I'm 6'3" and weigh 225, and Al is a lot bigger than I am. We shouldn't have any trouble with combative patients today
"Do you know where we're going?" I ask Al.
"Death Manor," he tells me and drives toward our destination. Dexter Manor is an enormous hi-rise located on the outskirts of the downtown area. The Providence Housing Authority has done their best keeping the place up, but it is very old and the years have taken their toll. Cockroaches and other crawly things can be seen running about despite the best efforts from the exterminators. The bugs are the least bothersome pests. Some of the people who live here don't follow the acceptable rules of a civilized society. The police are called to the building as often as we are. The Housecoat Brigade, a group of elderly residents that inhabit the hi-rises in Providence, and probably everywhere else, is conspicuously absent

from the halls. I don't think the other residents appreciate them, so I imagine they meet in secret and plan for the day that they will retake the building.

"How was your night?" I ask Al. He worked a callback on Rescue 3 last night and is on the last ten hours of a thirty-four.

"Shitty, how about yours?"

"Sucked."

"I got in yesterday morning and haven't stopped," he says. "This is something like my twentieth run in twenty-four hours. I hope things slow down or it's going to be a long day."

"Do you miss the ladder truck?" I ask.

"Nah, but this is getting ridiculous. I thought we were getting more rescues. When I came over to rescue the city promised one more truck that year, then another one the next. Two years have come and gone and nothing," says Al.

"I know, I did the same thing three years ago. I should have known better. We're just going to have to pace ourselves."

"That and drink a lot of coffee."

"Roger that."

"Every time I come back to Branch Avenue I feel like I've entered a time warp. Can you believe Wayne, Arthur and Kenny are still here?" I say. The first five years of my career were spent on Engine 2 at Branch Avenue. The crew is still the same, I am the one missing.

"They're going to retire here. I wouldn't know what to do if they left, they've become like family."

"That has to be the longest any group has stayed together. You guys are pretty lucky. The five years that I was on Engine 2 were the best years I had on the fire department. I don't think I've had a good belly laugh on the job since I left, and back then we had them every night," I say.

"It's not the same, but it's still pretty good. I'll probably stay there for a while."

We arrive on scene and find our patient waiting for us in the lobby, sitting on a bench and clutching his stomach. A woman who appears to be his wife is with him. She helps him to his feet and they both start to walk to the rescue. He is wearing Sergio Valente jeans, sneakers and a shocking pink polo shirt. A burgundy Members Only jacket completes the outfit. He takes his baseball cap off of his head as he enters the truck revealing a full head of gray frizzy hair. The woman who appears to be his wife gets in and sits next to him on the bench seat. Her bright blue pants and yellow sweater contrast nicely with the pink polo shirt. Easter has come early to the back of Rescue 3.

"What's the matter with him?" I ask.

"Pain, bad. Long time." She points to his abdominal area.

"Has he been throwing up?" I ask. She looks at me with a blank stare. I pantomime the act of vomiting, with sound effects, and she understands immediately what I'm talking about.

"Si!" She nods her head emphatically. "Three times."

"I didn't know you spoke Spanish," says Al.

"I've been taking classes."

Al gets the man's vital signs, tells them to me so I can document them on my report then gets in front to drive to Rhode Island Hospital. It is difficult to communicate with the two passengers in the back of my truck, so I fill out the report during the ride. It is only a mile away so the trip is a short one. We pull into the rescue bay and head to the triage area. I give my report to Katey who will be our Maitre'd this morning.

"Hi guys, how are you?" she asks.

"Better because you're here," I say.

"Fabulous," says Al.

"What have you got?" she asks.

"Fifty-two year old male complaining of abdominal pain for a 'long time.' He's been vomiting but there is a language barrier so I can't tell you much more than that."

"I think we can figure out what's wrong," Katey says and signs my report.

I often wonder what happens to the patients when I turn them over to the hospital staff. My contact with them is miniscule in comparison to their entire experience. The ride to the hospital is only the beginning; from there the real treatment begins.

"Do you have anything to do?" I ask Al as we head back to the station.

"No, I'm all set, how about you?"

"I've got to get to Venda to pick up some manicotti, and then visit my mother in the nursing home."

"How is she doing?"

"About the same. It's hard to believe that it's been eight years since she had the stroke."

"Does she recognize you when you visit?"

"Yeah, but she can't communicate or move. She's been on a feeding tube since the week after Christmas. I don't know how she has survived."

"My mother was in a coma for the last five years of her life," says Al. "I used to visit her all the time, so I know it's hard."

"It can be pretty depressing."

"Venda doesn't open until eleven, do you want to visit your mom first?"

"Let's go back to the station and try to get a little rest. We can do the other stuff after lunch.

"Good plan."

The radio is quiet on the way back to quarters. Maybe the rescue gods will be on our side for a change.

TEN

"It's a good thing you can write, because you can't cook worth a shit," says Wayne, with a big grin on his face, as I walk into the day room with Al.

"Maybe he'll make Oprah's Potatoes and we can all go home sick," says Arthur as he looks up from his newspaper. I made the potatoes ten years ago during one of my ill-fated creative forays in the kitchen and haven't heard the end of it. I was sure potato, honey and horseradish would be a great mix. Oprah was on TV at the time I was cooking so I named them "Oprah's Potatoes."

"Big talk for a one-meal chicken cooker," I say to Wayne, bringing to life another ghost from the past. "Chicken Oliveira" was the only meal Wayne ever made. Unlike Steve's Mexican Chicken, it was actually pretty good.

The rest of D group is sitting around, drinking coffee and figuring out the problems of the world. The letter to the editor that I wrote in yesterday's paper has been tacked to the bulletin board.

"Nice job, Morse," says the Captain of Engine 2, who was reading the letter when we walked in. He leaves it at that and takes his coffee to his office.

"Did Cheryl write that for you?" asks Kenny. "Because she's got the looks and the brains in your house."

"Every now and then I have a moment of clarity," I say.

"You haven't a clear thought in that big head of yours since you met Cheryl," says Wayne. "How's my girl feeling?" he asks. Every time I see these guys they ask about my wife. We were pretty tight early in my career, our wives and girlfriends all knew one another from the parties and cookouts we shared. I miss that camaraderie and wonder if I'll get it back before I retire. I don't see too much of it anymore and that is a pity.

"She's doing great, thanks for asking," I say.

"Make sure you tell her I said hello," says Wayne.

We pass the next hour catching up on things, and then the guys start the Saturday morning routine. Every Saturday the stove, oven and refrigerator are thoroughly cleaned. There is usually a smorgasbord left over from the week's meals. If not for the Saturday rule, things would get out of hand quickly. Men have a hard time throwing out perfectly good food.

On the apparatus floor, the drivers of Ladder 7, Engine 2, Rescue 3 and Battalion 3 have moved the vehicles onto the ramp so that the floor can be swept and washed. This is a Saturday routine that is being played out in every fire station in the city. Saturday is scrub out day. Period. Later, another firehouse tradition is in store; Saugy hot dogs, baked beans and snowflake rolls. Some stations veer from the course and have gotten healthy, eating chicken or salads, but the majority stick with tradition.

"I don't see the ping pong table, you must have hid it because you knew I was coming over." I say to Wayne when we return from the hospital. The apparatus floor is damp from the scrub out, the fresh smell of Spic-N-Span a welcome respite from the usual diesel and sewage. Unspeakable aromas and cat-sized rats come from a grate directly in front of Engine 2's bay. Closing the overhead doors helps a little but you can't keep unwanted things from getting in.

"Everybody knows there's no sense playing when they'll never win," says Wayne, acting nonchalant, but the gleam in his eye gives him away. He just can't pass up a good chance to give some poor soul a beating. If I had a nickel for every hour I spent trying to beat him, I'd have a lot of nickels. We played thousands of games over the years, I've only beaten him a handful of times. Every time it looks like I've got him, he gets all business and transforms himself into Forrest Gump. Little does he know that in the years I've been gone from the Branch Avenue Station, I've been training on my own table with a ping-pong master, another person I seldom beat, my brother, Bob. Cheryl surprised me on my birthday a few years ago, took me out to dinner. While we were enjoying ourselves, some of Danielle's friends went to Sears, picked up a professional grade table and set it up in our basement.

My brother, Bob has a table of his own and loves to beat his boys, Bobby and Danny. It's something we learned from our father, make the kids earn their victories. Ping Pong was big in our neighborhood when we were kids, the men of the neighborhood would gather at Dr. Carroll's garage when all of their "chores" were done, drink beer and play all afternoon. Every now and then one of the kids would get a chance at the table, only to be whooped by whoever was the champion at the time. They even had a trophy that they would pass around.

I don't know how he did it but brother Bob actually got pretty good. His job at the Adult Correctional Institute might have something to do with it, I'm sure the prisoners taught him a trick or two. We have been playing for years now, sometimes at my house, sometimes at his and are pretty evenly matched. He has more wins than I do, but he cheats.

"You gained a lot of weight since the last time," I say.

"And your head got bigger," he responds.

"Either your head is growing or your hair is shrinking, pretty shiny up top, I say."

"That's a solar panel for a love machine. Let's go, chump."

The table is stored in a room in back. We wheel it out, put it in the same place we spent so much time early in my career, at the bottom of the stairs, behind Engine 2. Some paddles and a few balls have been gathering dust in a corner. Fire station life is funny like that; pastimes come and go, then come again. A deck of cards upstairs has replaced the table, Hi-Lo Jack being the pastime of choice for now, I'm told. Maybe our game will resurrect the ping-pong table.

"Where's my paddle?" I ask. I had a favorite, soft on one side, hard on the other. The skin was wearing off and the handle missing some wood, probably from a flight across the station after one of Wayne's beatings.

"Don't matter, you ain't going to be hitting no balls back," says Wayne, a toothpick now at the corner of his mouth. He's all business now that he has a victim.

I grab a paddle, not my favorite but close.

"You want to warm up?"

"For you?" he says with a wicked grin. "Volley."

I toss the ball across the table and we are underway. We're both rusty but that will change. Back in the day we played so hard I developed tendonitis in my shoulder and elbow. He wins the volley.

"You sure you want to do this. Last chance to leave with some dignity."

"Serve," I say and a blur speeds past me.

"1-0."

Uh-oh. I have to go around Ladder 7 to find the ball, on the other side of the floor.

As soon as he gets the ball back it's past me again.

"You're gonna eat the next one," he says, not knowing I'm leading him into a false sense of security.

"2-0."

The next serve is easy to handle and a decent volley ensues. I leave a ball high and he slams it back.

"Told you. 3-0."

"Is that all you've got?"

It's amazing how a little ball creates a gust of wind when it flies by you.

"4-0."

I retrieve the ball, somewhere deep down a little doubt creeps in. I quickly crush it. I've learned a lot from Wayne over the years, a good lesson being to convince yourself you are unbeatable.

Wayne had been on the job for three years when I came along. Beneath his tough guy façade was a great guy, but it took me a while to figure that out. We came from different worlds, myself a middle class suburb outside of Providence, Wayne the heart of South Providence. A person's environment has a lot to do with how that person grows up, how they relate to the world around them, how they survive. Wayne's world, though only ten miles away from mine was altogether different. I lived in relative safety; Wayne learned early that life isn't always fair. A "blue-eyed black guy" on Broad Street stood out. He learned how to take care of himself, his bravado backed up with experience. He survived; some of his family did not.

"Eleven's a shutout," says Wayne, confident now, right where I want him.

"You can quit now before I start playing," I say, never letting him see me sweat. He shakes his head and blows another one past me.

Early Winter, 1992. A snowstorm blanketed the city with a foot of heavy, wet snow. On the ramp, seven of us manned the shovels, getting ready for the night's events. To move the snow you had to shovel it like dirt, no way it would be pushed out of the way. I was working like a madman, picking up a shovelful and dumping it thirty feet away on the side of the building then getting another load, over and over. I wasn't paying attention to the others, just content to move the snow my way, because my way was the right way, of course. I worked my way over to a mound of snow where everybody else had been dumping it, next to a fuel pump in front of the building. I didn't like the way it looked, it wasn't neat. I picked up a shovelful from the pile and dumped it next to the building.

"What the fuck are you doing?" Wayne asked, standing in front of me when I returned for another bite.

"Shoveling snow, what the fuck are you doing?"

"I'm watching an idiot make me work harder," he said.

"Worry about yourself," I said and thrust my shovel into the drift. Wayne kicked the bottom of the shovel, spilling the snow back where it came from.

"Pick it up." I said.

"Leave it there," he said.

"What's your problem?"

"You're my problem."

"What, do you live in a ghetto? It looks like shit in front of the door."

"What do you know about living in a ghetto?"

"I know I don't live in one. Go lay on the couch, I'll move it away from the door."

"You ain't moving nothing."

Things were at the breaking point when Chief Ronny Moura stepped in.

"Enough! Morse, get upstairs and start cooking!"

I had brought the ingredients for dinner in, it waited for somebody to throw it together. Sweet and hot sausage mixed with red skinned potatoes and onions, tossed with olive oil and some "secret" seasonings and a salad on the side. I didn't want to eat, I wanted to shovel snow. My way.

"Chief, I'll do it, it looks like shit piled up here."

"Shit gonna melt, you idiot," said Wayne, ready to knock my block off.

"Go," said the chief, pointing toward the stairs. I put my shovel down and walked away, convinced the chief was going to make Wayne move the snow. It wasn't the result I was looking for, I didn't want anybody fighting my battles for me, but I took it.

Things cooled down, a peaceful coexistence ensued and we moved on. I noticed later that the snow pile was right where Wayne and everybody else had piled it.

Eventually, the snow melted.

"0-5"

I threw the ball a foot in the air, sliced under it and watched Wayne's shocked expression as it sailed past him.

"1-5"

This time I put some topspin on the ball, Wayne almost caught up.

"2-5"

I tried a little razzle-dazzle sidespin and missed the table.

"What did I tell you about beating yourself? You ain't learned nothin'."

"2-6"

He hit my serve back and we battled for a while, I eventually snuck one past him.

"3-6. Is that sweat I see on the dome?" I asked, giving the ball a whack. He whacked it back, right past me.

"Who's sweatin' now, chump?"

"3-7, your serve."

Spring, 1993

I had bid a spot on Engine 2, this was my first week driving. The driver of the truck, also known as the chauffer is responsible for getting the crew to the incident quickly and safely, apparatus placement on scene, the proper running of the vehicle, all of the tools and EMS supplies and most important, the pump. This particular morning Engine 2 was detailed *from the Branch Avenue Station in the North End to South Providence. Our job was to be available for calls while the fire companies from Broad Street were conducting a fire extinguisher drill at one of the fuel companies that inhabit the Port of Providence. Kenny, the officer in charge that day was working overtime and had no idea this was my first week driving the engine. Wayne and Arthur occupied the rear jump seats, each with their own particular set of duties for whatever call we were sent on.*

Halfway through the drill the truck radio sparked to life;

"Attention Engine 2, Engine 11, Engine 3, Special Hazards, Ladder1, Ladder 8 and Rescue 1, respond to 151 Washington Avenue for a fire on the second floor, reports of trapped occupants."

We roared out of the drill yard toward the fire. I saw smoke coming from over the tree line about a mile from our position.

"All companies responding to 151 Washington be advised, there is an infant on the third floor and a handicapped male in a wheelchair on the first."

I made the truck go faster. Behind me Wayne and Arthur were "getting dressed," putting on their turnout gear, no easy task in a speeding truck with limited room to move. Kenny did the same while answering the radio.

We were first in. I was responsible for the positioning of the apparatus and the pump. I turned the engine down Washington Avenue and saw flames shooting from a second floor balcony. Cars were parked on both sides of the street leaving just enough room to squeeze through.

"Go fifty feet past it," said Kenny, calmly, referring to the burning house. Ladder 5, right behind us needed room to set up the aerial ladder. I stopped the truck, Kenny went in looking for victims, Wayne and Arthur went to the rear and grabbed a hand line and started the process of stretching it into the front door of the fire building. Ladder 5 stopped

behind me, two members immediately went to into the house, and two got the ladder ready.

At this point I had Kenny, Wayne and Arthur inside the burning building, an infant on the third floor, a handicapped man in a wheelchair on the first, and two firefighters on the roof.

"Charge my line!" came the muffled order from Wayne who had found the fire.

I put the truck in pump by putting the engine in neutral, hitting a switch that transferred the power to the pump, then shifting back into drive. The red throttle handle on the pump panel controlled the pump's RPM, I needed it to get to 150 psi to get the right pressure to the nozzle. I turned the throttle, heard the engine strain and expected the gauge to show something. It stayed at zero. Smoke came from under the truck. Engine 10 had joined the fight, backing up Engine 2.

"Charge Engine 10's line!" came from the radio. I had nothing to give them. All of my training led me to this point. I felt the crushing weight of the responsibility for all of the lives depending on me. I turned the throttle higher, still no movement on the gauge. The truck jumped a foot forward. I froze. The officer of Engine 10 screamed for water, I tried harder but nothing worked. At the depths of despair, just when I thought the pressure of the situation would crush me, Wayne appeared from the back of the engine, walked over to the pump panel and figured out the problem.

"You're not in pump."

It clicked. When I flipped the pump switch on from inside the truck, the adrenaline was so high I probably switched it back off with out realizing it. The truck was in drive. It's a miracle it didn't run down the street and kill somebody. Thankfully the maxi-brake held. Wayne opened the cab door, put the truck in neutral, stepped over to the pump panel, throttled down, then put the truck in pump, throttled up to 150 psi, opened the gates for Engine 2 and Engine 10's lines and told me,

"Go fight some fire."

He pumped for the rest of the incident, I found Arthur, we eventually put the fire out. The handicapped man and the infant were saved, everybody survived. After the fire, while we were picking up I expected Wayne to start torturing me. Instead, he explained what I had done wrong, even tried to give me an out by suggesting the truck malfunctioned. Some of the other guys were not so forgiving. I learned a lot that day, lessons about pumping, grace under pressure, and that I loved Wayne like a brother.

Wayne is the only person I've met whose skull is thicker than my own. He sees things his way, I see them my way, neither one of us will ever admit the other is right. I have come to respect the man and understand that the way he goes about the job, while different from the way I do things, is just as effective when looking at the big picture. The fires go out, the patients are given the best care and the station is maintained. If anything I have learned to relax a little, and am better for it.

"7 serving 3"

The game went on, an up and down battle, both players giving it their all. It was tied at twenty when the bell tipped.

ELEVEN

0934 hrs (9:34 a.m.)

"Rescue 3 and Engine 7; respond to 268 Benefit Street for an elderly male who has fallen down the stairs,"

We put down the paddles; I went for the Rescue, Wayne for the couch.

We leave the station and turn left toward Benefit Street. When Providence was an industrial powerhouse, factory workers and their families inhabited the homes that line the historic street. Textile mills and factories were abundant nearby, most of which have since been destroyed by fire. Some of the mills have been converted to living space or offices but nobody is making much of anything these days in Providence, the manufacturing base has been shipped overseas. The Providence Preservation Society saw the value of the old homes that had been subdivided and turned into tenements long before developers and real estate professionals did and insisted the homes be preserved. Rather than let the area be redeveloped or demolished, the buildings were restored. We now have the finest cohesive collection of restored 18th and early

19th century architecture in the United States right at our doorstep. The "Mile of History" is one of the most prolific, vibrant parts of the city. Reproduction gas street lamps illuminate the area at night; you can imagine yourself walking in the footsteps of Edgar Allen Poe who spent his later years in Providence courting a reputable widow, Sarah Whitman at the Providence Athenaeum, the fourth oldest private library in the country.

The guys from Engine 9 are inside the historic home; their truck parked about thirty feet past the doorway leaving room for the rescue. We pull the stretcher from the back of the rig; place a long spine board on top and walk in, passing a cast iron boot scraper that has been there for centuries.

An elderly couple sits on a couch in the front room. Bob Cataldo from the 9's gives me the story.

"He was trying to help his wife up the stairs with the laundry basket, she was raising it up to the balcony, he leaned too far and fell over the balcony and right on top of her."

"No way," I say, shocked that the people are not more seriously hurt. I walk over to the stairs, a balcony with a three foot railing is at the head of the stairway which has a landing about ten feet down, then another seven or eight steps.

"Way," says Bob.

"Are you folks okay?" I ask the gray haired couple sitting next to each other on the couch. The man is crooked, rubbing his lower back, his wife sits straight, but has a laceration and bump on her forehead.

"I'm fine, I'm worried about her," the man says.

"I'm okay, I'm worried about him," she replies.

"I'm worried about both of you. I can't believe you two walked away after that fall. You must be pretty tough."

"Sixty years of marriage will do that," they say at the same time, and then smile at each other.

"We're going to get you to the hospital, just bear with us, I want to get you immobilized on a backboard for the ride."

"I know how that goes," says the man, "just a few months ago we were in a car accident on Academy Avenue, I went through it then. It's a good thing I did, the doctors at Miriam Hospital said the EMT's saved me from being paralyzed, I had a broken neck."

"I thought you two looked familiar," I said, "that was me! A hit and run driver sideswiped you and ran you into a utility pole. If I remember correctly, you were worried about your wife."

"He's the one that ended up in the hospital for a week," she said, reaching over to hold her husband's hand. "There was nothing wrong with me."

With help from the engine company we "package" our patients for the ride to the hospital. I still can't believe these two elderly people had two traumatic incidents in the last month and managed to tell the tale. From the look of things, no serious harm was done by the fall, which is truly amazing. First, a fall of ten feet can be serious at any age, being eighty increases the chance of broken bones or worse. Second, having a two-hundred pound man fall on you from ten feet has its share of complications.

We ride down Benefit Street toward the hospital, my patients, together for better and worse under my care again.

TWELVE

I head to the privacy of my office and decide to test the waters at home. I take my phone from my top pocket and plunge. Cheryl answers on the first ring.

"Hello."

"Hey babe, how are you?"

"Fine."

"What's going on?"

"Nothing."

"Are you going to give me one word answers all day?"

"I'm not playing any games, I'm just tired. You didn't really do anything wrong, I've just got a lot on my mind."

"Me too. What time is dinner tomorrow?"

"I'm going to try for three. You should have had enough rest by then."

"I'll be fine."

"I know. Call me later."

"Alright. Love you, bye."

"Love you too."

Lukewarm. It seems there may be hope. I want to go to Venda now, but I don't want to wake Al up if he is sleeping. We have to take care of each other. However, if I don't come through with the goods, I'll never hear the end of it. The couch is irresistible and sucks me in.

1157 hrs. (11:57 a.m.)

"Rescue 3 and Engine 2, a still alarm."

My eyes pop open and I'm instantly awake. I don't have to wait long for the rest of the transmission.

"Rescue 3 and Engine 2, respond to 74 Ledge Street for a seven-year old who is unconscious."

"This kid doesn't know the meaning of unconscious," I say to Al as we head out the door behind Engine 2. I have responded to hundreds of emergency calls for unconscious people only to find them wide-awake when I get there. I don't know why people say that the person they are calling for is unconscious; maybe they think we'll get there faster. Of course, there is always the chance that the person actually is unconscious, in that case we will be ready and respond accordingly.

We follow Engine 2 as they make their way over Rt. 95 and into the north end of the city. Single-family homes are mixed with multi-unit properties, some well kept, the majority dumps. Twenty years ago this was a respectable area. The older residents tell of how it used to be when I get them in the back of the truck. With sadness in their voices they tell me about the neighborhood before the trash moved in. I am not a fan of generalization, but it is hard to ignore the facts. I see some homes meticulously kept, and others suffering from neglect and can feel the old folks' pain. Nobody wants to see the street where they lived and raised their families lose its dignity, but that is the picture they see when they look out of their windows.

Engine 2 pulls past the house on Ledge Street and Al pulls Rescue 3 in front. As soon as the vehicle stops, a seven year old boy walks out the front door and lets himself into the back of the rescue.

"Can you find out what that kid is doing?" I ask Al. He goes to the back of the truck and I head to the front door. The guys from Engine 2 follow me in.

"What's going on over here?" I ask a thirtyish guy dressed in his pajamas.

"He's sick. The hospital didn't do nothing so we're sending him back."

"What are you talking about?" I ask.

"The rescue took him to Hasbro last night because he was puking. He's still puking today so we're sending him back."

"Are you nuts?" I ask. He looks at me with a blank stare. The place is filthy. A picture of Robert De Niro adorns the front door, the only decent item in the entire place.

"Where is his mother?" I ask.

"Getting dressed. She'll be there in a minute."

I cannot believe the audacity of this guy. The people of this city truly believe we are at their beck and call. Not only is he abusing the 911 system today, he did it last night as well.

"Why don't you take him to the hospital yourself?" I ask.

"I don't have a car."

"Why don't you get a car?"

Just then the boy's mother comes out of a rear bedroom. She looks frail and exhausted. I tell myself that nothing is going to change by trying to make these people see the error of their ways.

"Let's go," I say to the mother. "You guys are all set," I tell the members of Engine 2. This surprises none of them; they've seen it all before.

Al is waiting in the back of the rescue. He has made a friend. He has the sick boy lying on the stretcher covered with a giant stack of blankets he got out of one of the storage compartments.

"What's this?" I ask.

"He said he was cold."

"Not anymore," I say as the boy laughs heartily. I put the mother on the bench seat and get ready to go.

"Why are you going back to the hospital?" I ask.

"He's still sick," she says.

"He's going to be sick here or at the hospital. Why don't you keep him at home, put him to bed and give him some soup?"

"We don't have any soup," she says. I give up. Al has taken the boy's vital signs and temperature and has found them to be normal.

"Hasbro?' he says as he leaves the back of the truck.

"Code C." I say and get ready to take down the boy's information.

THIRTEEN

"I have got to go see my mom," I say to Al as we leave Hasbro. Our patient has been checked in at the triage desk, much to the chagrin of the ER nurses. There is nothing they can do for the boy that wasn't done last night. The boy's mother had the state sponsored medical card ready when she went to the desk. I wonder if she would have been so quick to bring the boy back to the hospital if she was paying for the visit rather than the taxpayers. The health care situation in this country is out of control. People are paying incredible amounts of money for healthcare, or going without. The poor are covered and the rich aren't concerned. The folks in the middle continue to bear the brunt of keeping the country afloat

"How about after lunch," Al says. "I'm starving."

"Me too. Let's eat."

As expected, Saugy hot dogs, baked beans and snowflake rolls await us as we return to Branch Avenue. Saugys are a local delicacy. They are made only in Rhode Island and have been a firehouse tradition for years. I take three, only after telling everyone that there are eighteen grams of fat in each one, fill the rest of my plate with beans and top it off with three snowflake rolls. I cut the hotdogs in half lengthwise, then the other way so that they will fit inside the square rolls. Some catsup, mustard and relish and I'm good to go.

The rest of the guys have finished, they began eating at noon, and have cleaned the kitchen and are clearing out. The morning's work is done. For the rest of the day there is nothing for them to do but wait for the bell to tip. With any luck, it will be quiet.

As soon as lunch is finished we head to my mother's nursing home, only a few minutes from the station. When I had to find a place for her, Berkshire Place had just opened. The close proximity to the Branch Avenue fire station helped me decide where best to place her. My mother was one of the first residents there and is well known and liked by the staff. The home has done a great job with her care, for which I am grateful.

Al parks the truck in the fire lane and I get out and go to the third floor to visit. I walk into her room and see that she is sleeping. I don't want to wake her, but this is the last time I will see her until next week and I want to wish her a happy Easter. I used to bring ice cream or some other treat, but her health has deteriorated and she can no longer swallow without choking. The machine makes a clicking sound every second as the bag full of nourishment goes from the tube into my mother's body, giving her no satisfaction but sustaining her life. I don't know how she keeps the will to live. I speak to her gently and she opens her eyes. They are as clear and bright as they were before the stroke, full of intelligence. She lifts her good arm, caresses my face and smiles with the half of her face that isn't paralyzed. I take her hand, hold it and wait for the radio to send me on another run; there is nothing else I can do. After ten minutes I am called away.

1346 hrs. (2:46 p.m.)

"Rescue 3 a still alarm."

"Bye Mom, happy Easter."

"*Rescue three and Engine 2, respond to University Heights for an elderly man with difficulty breathing.*"

"Rescue 3 responding."

"How is she?" Al asks as I get into the truck.
"Same."
We make our way to University Heights as Neil Young sings "Old Man."
University Heights is about five minutes from our present location. Engine 2 will be there in one. I wait for their transmission with the radio mike in my hand, tapping along with Neil's acoustic guitar.

"Engine 2 to fire alarm, we have a sixty-one year old male, conscious and alert complaining of slight difficulty breathing. We're assessing vitals now and putting him on 02."
"Rescue 3 received."

I can see the flashing lights from Engine 2 as we turn into the University Heights Apartments. Standing next to the engine with a nasal canula attached to his face and dressed in a brown leather trench coat is our patient. He sees the rescue and makes his way toward us. He doesn't appear to be in much distress.
"He's fine, some kids were giving him a hard time and he ran away from them now he can't catch his breath," says Captain Crowley.
"I was walking like I do every morning. These kids around here are no good," he says. "I stopped to have a cigarette and the little pricks tried to rob me. I didn't run away, I walked after telling them the fuck off. I started feeling dizzy so I called 911."

"Get in the truck," I say to the man. "Thanks, Cap, you guys are all set." The engine company heads back to the station and the rescue appears to be heading to the hospital.

Al has the man seated on the bench seat and is assessing his vital signs.

"120/60, pulse 70 and pulsox 99%. You're in better shape than I am," he tells the man.

"What is your name?" I ask and get the report out.

"Daniel Webster. I have to go to Miriam. Do you think I'll make in time for lunch?"

"Why do you have to go to the hospital?" I ask.

"I feel dizzy. I was there on Wednesday and they didn't do anything but give me some pills."

"Did you take the pills?"

"I don't believe in no pills."

Sometimes the absurdity of what I do to make a living is too much. Runs like these try my patience. I find out that Daniel is on disability because of depression. He hasn't worked in twenty years. Today's trip to the hospital, including the three-hundred dollar two-mile cab ride will cost the taxpayers more than a thousand dollars. I hope the lunch is worth it.

Miriam is full, with patients lined up in the hallway. We have Daniel seated in a wheelchair and are waiting for the charge nurse to take our report. We could be waiting a while. I see Bernie is in charge of triage today so I don't expect to be giving my report any time soon. Al has retrieved a nasal canula from the supply room and has decided to wait for me in the truck. I note the time of arrival on my report and begin to wait. Eventually, Bernie comes over.

"What have you got?" he asks.

"Sixty-one year old male complaining of dizziness, vitals are stable, history of depression. He was here on Wednesday, was prescribed some pills but doesn't believe in them." I hand the report to Bernie who signs it and walks away. He has been doing this a lot longer than me and has seen it all so I don't take his demeanor personally. At times he can actually be pleasant. From the look of things, the hospital will be diverting soon. When an area hospital has no more beds they can close the facility to rescues. An announcement is made over the air that the diverting hospital is diverting. Miriam is usually the first of the area hospitals to use the diversion plan. If two other hospitals follow suit, all area hospitals are forced open.

"Let's go to Venda," I say to Al when I get beck into the truck. The rescue gods have other plans.

FOURTEEN

1445 hrs. (2:45 p.m.)

"Rescue 3 are you available?" comes from the truck radio.

"Should I lie?" I ask Al.

"One small lie leads to bigger ones."

"Thanks Dad. Rescue 3 in service, what have you got?"

"Respond to the Providence Place for a seizure in the food court."

"On the way."

Al hits the lights and siren and we are on our way to the mall.

"Head to the south side," I tell Al.

"The north side is easier," he says.

"I want to go through the south side." I say.

"Then we'll have to walk twice as far."

"It's not that far. Last week I saw a girl Brittany's age fall from the escalator on the north side, I want to avoid that scene if at all possible."

"You had that?" says Al.

"Me and Tim Kelly. Ladder 4 was first on scene.

"What happened?"

"I was working overtime on Rescue 5. It was pretty quiet until about midnight, and then things got crazy. We had just gotten back in quarters from another run when a call came in for a female who had fallen at the mall. We followed Ladder 4 there. As we made our way to the scene things just felt wrong. When I got to the stairs I saw her, and I knew right away she wasn't going to make it. She was so still, and a pool of blood was forming around her head. Mall security was there but didn't know what to do. I asked one of them what happened and he told me she fell from the escalator. I looked up and saw the only place she could have fallen from and landed where she did was at least forty feet up."

"What did you do?"

"It took a while to get the stretcher to her, by that time the guys from Ladder 4 had done an assessment. She didn't have a pulse and wasn't breathing. Johnny Morgan tried to put a collar on her and felt the back of her head was soft. We put her on a board, got her on a stretcher and into the truck. Somebody started a line, I tried but couldn't intubate her and we got rolling. We ran a trauma code on the way to the ER and had a pulse when we got there."

"That was pretty good," says Al.

"Not good enough. I was hoping we saved her, but when I asked the doctor later how she was doing he told me that she was being kept alive for organ donation."

"That's pretty harsh."

"I thought so too, but the reality is we kept her going long enough for her parents and fiancé to say goodbye. Whether or not she heard is anybody's guess."

"Not much of a victory."

"No kidding, but it's better than nothing. A couple of days later I read her obituary in the paper. She was about to graduate college and become a teacher. She had a son and was getting married this summer. Do you know what I remember most about the whole thing?"

"No, what."

"Next to where she fell was a stuffed Spider Man doll. She had been at Dave and Buster's and probably won it and couldn't wait to give it to her son. I saw it when we were wheeling her out; that and the pool of blood where her head had been. I wonder if the stain is still there."

Al pulls the truck in front of the south entrance.

"A little extra walking won't kill us," he says.

"Thanks."

Mall security meets us at the door and escorts us through the labyrinth behind the pretty façade. The management likes to keep us out of sight for as long as possible. After a few minutes and an elevator ride, we are allowed entry to the food court. It is teeming with people. Alone at a table off to the side sits a middle-aged woman drinking a beverage through a straw from a plastic cup. Security points her out.

"What happened to her?" I ask the guard.

"I don't know, they told me to take you to her, that's all."

"Thanks."

We keep the stretcher out of sight and walk over to our patient.

"Hello," says Al.

"How are you feeling?" I add.

"Fine, I don't need any help and I'm not going anywhere," she tells us.

"That's fine with us, but somebody called and said that you had a seizure," I tell her.

"I may have had a little one, but I'm fine now."

She appears to have a developmental disability. Her day at the mall is likely something that she looks forward to and I don't want to take that away. However, if she did have a seizure, another could be imminent and she could get hurt.

"How did you get here?" I ask.

"The bus."

"Is there anybody here with you?"

"Nope."

"Do you have a history of seizures?"

"I do but I take my medication every day," she states emphatically.

"I'm going to ask you some simple questions to determine if you are able to make good decisions," I tell her. "Do you know what day it is?"

"Nope. Doesn't matter." She has a point.

"Do you know the date?"

"Stupid question. If I don't care what day it is why should I care about the date."

"Got me. Do you know who is President?"

"Bill Clinton," she says. That is good enough for me. I am a threat to her independence so she has no intention of cooperating. She has shown me some spark and a quick wit. I am sure she will be fine.

"You're doing better than me," I tell her. "If you feel a seizure coming on or have any pain anywhere don't wait until it's too late, call for help," I say.

"Have a nice day," she says and gets up and walks away.

FIFTEEN

"Do you need anything while we're here?" I ask Al as we make our way back to the rescue. This time we go through the main part of the mall.

"I'm all set, let's get a coffee and head over to Venda."

"I'm buying," I say and we walk through the mall while pushing the stretcher. People don't give us a second look as we pass, they are too busy shopping, or in the case of the teen population scoping out the opposite sex. The two old rescue guys are doing the same, only not as blatantly, and the opposite sex isn't looking back. I feel a vibration from my pants pocket and know it could only be one thing.

"Hello."

"What's up?" Cheryl asks.

"Nothing, just getting through the day. I had to go to the mall for a seizure."

"Did you go past where that girl fell?"

"No, we went the other way."

"You have to face it sooner or later."

"I know, I prefer later."

"You know what's best, just don't wait too long."

I have a habit of avoiding places where tragedies occur until I've made peace with my memories. The girl who fell off of the escalator and the Spider Man doll she lost is still bouncing around in my head, and probably will be for a long time to come. That run was horrendous and I've yet to come to terms with it. It helps to talk about what happened, and I have at length with my wife, but it still is going to take more time for the painful images to stop haunting me. The department offers a critical incident stress debriefing which is a very effective way to handle the grief that comes with the job but I chose to deal with this one on my own. The people on the debriefing team do a great job and are trained to help emergency personnel get through the muddy waters we sometimes find ourselves drowning in. Had I called for assistance, everybody involved in the incident would have met at one of the stations and talked about what happened. It really does help to deal with the conflicting emotions we all feel after witnessing the horrific things we see, and to see that the people we work with feel the same way makes the sorrow easier to bear.

The night the girl fell to her death I was on the end of a thirty-eight hour shift. Her's was my thirtieth run in that time span. I was too tired to talk and opted to try to get some rest instead of staying awake talking. Instead of resting, we responded to three more runs before I was relieved at seven the next morning. I should have spent the time talking, but it was too late.

"Thanks for worrying about me," I say.

The silly fighting between us seems to have subsided and I want to keep the good vibe flowing.

"I got the manicotti."

"Great, my mother loves it. I didn't mean to get on you about not picking it up, I just get frustrated being stuck in this house."

"I know, I don't mind helping out."

Al and I have made it back to the rescue. He has been eavesdropping; I can tell by the way he is shaking his head.

"Call me later."

"Love you, bye."

"Love you too."

I put the phone back in my pocket and look at Al.

"What's the matter with you?" I ask.

"Do you have the manicotti?"

"No, but we're going over there now."

"What if we don't make it," he asks.

"We'll make it, it's right up the road," I say as we get in and head toward Federal Hill.

It's almost 3:30 and the traffic has eased a little as we head over to the store. Lunch is over, dinner has not begun and the restaurants and cafés are nearly empty. As we get closer to our destination I feel my stomach sink. The lights are out at Venda, the doors are locked, and there will be no manicotti at the Morse house tomorrow.

"What did I tell you about little lies?" Al asks as I sit in my seat and will the store to be open. I'm in no mood for his righteousness.

"I was lying when I said I liked you."

"Ow! That hurt," says Al with a laugh that doesn't sound even a little painful.

"I'm doomed."

"Just tell her the store was closed," Al offers.

"It's not that, it's that I told her I had them. I know! I'll tell her I forgot them in the refrigerator."

"Bigger lies."

"What would I do without you," I ask.

"Tell bigger and better lies I guess."

We ride around the area for a while then decide to get back to quarters. If we don't get any more runs, Al will go home and I'll get back to Rescue 1 and relieve Tim.

"Rescue 3 a still alarm."

1708 hrs (5:08 p.m.)

"Rescue 3; respond to 184 Lydia Street for a pregnant female with abdominal pain."

"Rescue 3, responding."

We are only a few blocks away from Lydia Street; Al hits the lights and siren and gets us there in less than a minute. We pull the truck in front of a triple decker that looks fairly well kept and see a small woman running down the front steps and over to the truck. Before either of us can open the doors she approaches.

"Hurry up, my sister is bleeding."

"Get out of the way," I say, and she moves away from my door.

"Where is the blood coming from?" I ask as we make our way to the front door. Al has retrieved the stair chair from the rear compartment and is right behind us.

"From her private parts," she says as we walk into the house. Our patient is sitting on a couch in a sparsely furnished room, her skin pale and damp. Al takes one look and sets up the chair; there is no way this girl is walking.

"Are you in any pain?" I ask. Her sister starts to answer.

"Let her talk." I say.

"I'm thirty-two weeks pregnant," she says, "an hour ago I started feeling some cramping, then I noticed I was bleeding."

"Take her to the hospital," her sister demands. We ignore her for now, I'm trying to get a history and have every intention of taking her to the hospital as quickly as possible.

"Do you have any other children?" I ask.

"Yes, two. I also had a miscarriage a few years ago."

"Okay, we're going to get going," I say as Al and I pick her up, put her into the stair chair, secure the straps and carry her to the truck. Her sister comes with us and insists on riding in the back.

"Start an IV and get going," she says as soon as we are settled in the back of the rescue.

"Do you want to stay back here?" I ask.

"Just do your job," she says. Al and I are too tired to argue, and the patient needs an IV and immediate medical assistance. Al gets the IV on the first try, while I take her vital signs. The girl is the perfect patient, her sister the total opposite. I want to get her to Women and Infants as quickly as possible, something is wrong. She needs to be seen in a hospital and may end up in the operating room.

"BP 90/60, Pulse 120, I tell Al. Her vitals are not good and he knows it, with nothing more needed to be said he heads to the front of the truck and wastes no time getting to the hospital. I monitor my patient -her name is Po Ling - while speeding toward the ER, and phone them on the way.

"ER Triage," says the R.N. on the phone.

"Hello, Providence Rescue 3 calling. I've got a twenty-five year old patient, thirty-two weeks pregnant with her third child, one miscarriage with heavy vaginal bleeding. She is hypotensive at this time with a rapid pulse and experiencing abdominal pain. We have her on oxygen, an IV established ETA five minutes."

"See you then," the nurse hangs up the phone. I'm sure that she is informing the ER staff of our situation and they are getting a room ready for our arrival.

I get a non-rebreather from the compartment over my seat, turn the oxygen tank on and set the flow to ten liters per minute. I fill the reservoir by holding a finger over a valve at the bottom of the mask, pull back the elastic band, and then place the device over Po's face.

"This is oxygen," I tell her, "it will help you and the baby." She smiles, sits back on the stretcher and closes her eyes. I can see signs of pain all over the delicate features of her face.

"I'm sorry I've been so mean," her sister says.

"That's all right. You're under a lot of stress, I understand," I say.

"Will she be okay?"

I want to lie and tell her everything will be fine. The problem is, I don't know how this is going to turn out. There could be a number of things going wrong right now, and don't have a clue what they are.

"Right now her vital signs are a little irregular but she is stable. When we get to the hospital we'll know more."

The truck stops in front of the emergency room door and Al opens the back doors letting the chilly air into the back. I help Po's sister out the side door and Al wheels the stretcher out the back. As expected, the ER staff has a room ready for us. We head back to the treatment area, and then transfer our patient from our stretcher to the hospital's. The triage nurse signs my report and I have nothing more to do with Po or her sister. I hope everything turns out okay, but it looks like she is having a miscarriage. I plan to come back later to check the status of the baby and her mom. For now, they are receiving the best possible care, and all I can do is wish them well.

SIXTEEN

We're leaving the Woman and Infants parking lot when the radio transmits.

"Engine 13, respond with a Cranston rescue to the corner of Thurbers and Eddy for a woman unconscious with multiple stab wounds."

Eddy and Thurbers is close to our location. I key the mic.

"Rescue 3 to fire alarm, we're clearing Woman and Infants and can respond with Engine 13."

"Roger, Rescue 3, at 1748.

Al's shift should have been over forty-eight minutes ago and I have to get back to Rescue 1 to relieve Tim. A woman may be dying on the sidewalk. It is not her fault that the city has chosen to ignore the obvious need for more rescues. She is fortunate that she wasn't stabbed ten minutes ago, we would not have been able to help. I'll put Al in for an hour's overtime, Tim will have to wait.

1748 hrs. (5:48 p.m.)

This is why we're here. The girl we just brought to Women and Infants and the lady possibly dying from multiple stab wounds are what keep me going. All of the nonsense and free taxi rides to the hospital are forgotten when a real emergency comes in. When I was fighting fires I felt a similar adrenaline rush as we sped toward our destination. The lights and sirens let people know we're coming through as we push our way through traffic to the aid of the injured woman.

"Engine 13 to fire alarm, we have a thirty year-old female semi-conscious with a stab wound to the upper chest and another to the lower abdomen, controlling bleeding and getting vitals."

"Rescue 3, received and on the scene."

A crowd of police, news reporters and curious bystanders has gathered around the wounded woman. Al pulls the truck as close to her as he can. She is lying on her back struggling with the members of Engine 13. The police are trying to get the crowd under control, there is a lot of yelling and finger pointing going on. Al gets the stretcher from the back of the truck, stopping to get a long board from the rear compartment. He puts it on top of the stretcher and we bring it next to the victim and lower it. Captain Healy gives me another report.

"She got into a fight with her friend who pulled out a four inch knife and stabbed her a couple of times. She says she can't breath. We're trying to get a collar on her but she's fighting us."

"Thanks. I need a driver and two of your guys in the back."

"Let's get her on the board," I say to Al. Steve, Jay and Art from Engine 13 help him.

"What is your name?" I ask the patient.

"Tanisha. That bitch stabbed me," she says, sounding more shocked than angry.

"She stabbed you twice actually. Tanisha, I have to put this collar around your neck in case your spine was injured okay?"

"Go ahead."

"Thanks. Now we're going to put you on this board. It's a little uncomfortable, but that is what the hospital wants us to do."

"I can't breath." She says as we move her onto the longboard and lift her onto the stretcher. She is still a little feisty but is running out of energy. Art has filled a non-rebreather from Engine 13's portable 02 tank and puts the mask over Tanisha's face. She immediately pulls it off and repeats,

"I can't breath!"

"This is oxygen, give it a few seconds, it will help you," I tell her. She settles down but her breathing is too rapid. We get her into the truck and get to work.

"I need a large bore IV, an EKG, vitals and we need to cut these clothes off."

"You ain't cuttin my clothes!" says Tanisha, ripping the oxygen mask from her face.

"Sorry, I'll try not to ruin them," I tell her. I get her out of her jacket but have to cut the shirt and bra. Al puts the leads on her then covers her with a sheet. He puts the mask back on without much of a fight from her because she is slipping into unconsciousness. She has two stab wounds to her upper torso, one on her upper left chest and the other on the lower abdomen. The hospital is two minutes away. The monitor shows her rhythm as sinus tachycardia. I run a strip, put a stethoscope on and listen to her lungs.

"Let's go," I say.

Jay and Steve are with me in the back of the truck, Art is driving and the Captain is following in Engine 13.

I pick up the truck's cell phone and hit the automatic call for Rhode Island Hospital.

"Rhode Island ER."

"Providence Rescue 3 calling."

"Hello Providence, what have you got."

"Thirty year-old female, unconscious with two stab wounds, one to the upper chest, the other to the lower left abdominal quadrant, diminished lung sounds on the left side, pulsox 89% with hi-flow 02, BP 110/60 with a pulse of 120. We'll have an IV established when we get there in about a minute."

"See you then."

While I talked to the trauma nurse over the phone, Al established an IV and Steve got Tanisha's vital signs. I placed a defibrillator pad over the chest wound and secured it on three sides allowing excessive intrathoracic pressure to escape, preventing a condition called tension pneumothorax. If this occurs, the patient is in a serious, life threatening condition and needs decompression, something I am not permitted to do. We have her immobilized, a cervical collar applied and placed on a backboard. I can feel from the bumps in the road that the ER is thirty seconds away. Seven minutes have elapsed since we arrived on scene.

A trauma team has assembled and is waiting for us in Trauma Room 2. We wheel Tanisha through the triage area and into trauma alley where she is transferred by us from our stretcher onto a trauma stretcher. The trauma team is waiting for my report.

"Thirty year old female, stab wound from a four inch knife to the upper left chest, diminished lung sounds, left side. Last pulsox 92% with fifteen liters, another stab wound from the same weapon lower left abdominal quadrant, abdomen feels hard on palpation, blood pressure initially 110/60, it was 98/60 upon arrival, IV access sixteen gauge, left AC.

The trauma team has heard what they need from me; I'm no longer necessary. The guys from Engine 13 are standing outside the door waiting to see the outcome. Al needs some help putting the truck back together so I go and help him. Later, I'll find out how Tanisha made out. I'll be here all night.

"What a finish," says Al as we get the truck ready for the next run. He looks completely exhausted, but I know, like me he feels exhilarated. Tanisha was knocking on heavens door twenty minutes ago, and we played a huge part in saving her life.

"It's not over yet, we still have to get back to Branch Avenue," I say as we leave the hospital parking lot.

"Don't jinx us," says Al. We ride back in silence, satisfied.

PART III

SATURDAY NIGHT

SEVENTEEN

Saturday Night. I'm going in sleep deprived and cranky with a long night ahead. I remember a time when Saturday nights were considered "date night," with Friday more of the "party" time. Here in the Capitol City, Saturday nights are a no holds barred slugfest. I try not to jinx myself with negative thoughts, but I've found that no matter how positive my outlook, Saturday nights in Providence are a night in a torture chamber.

So far, we're off to a great start with the double stabbing and without a doubt things will spiral downhill from here. Years of experience have taught me to expect the worst. For now though, nothing can touch me. I have time to relish the peace, quiet and solitude the old wagon offers during the trip back to the Allens Avenue Fire Station. My car is my fortress; nobody can touch me here.

There have been times that the solitary ride wasn't so great.

Early Winter, 1992.

"Attention Engines 12, 2, 7, ladders 3 and 7, Special Hazards, Rescue 3 and Car 23, respond to the corners of Dorothy and Charles for a cave-in with a man trapped."

This is what I lived for, what I trained for, what I would do for the next twenty years at least; rescue people. I hit the pole while the echo from the loudspeaker still filled the station, stepped into my bunker gear and climbed into Ladder 7's tiller cab. Steve Rocchio was already in the driver's seat, Lieutenant Healy was "getting dressed," and almost ready to climb into the officer's seat. I squeezed into the tiny seat in the tiller man's compartment, and immediately pressed the button that enabled the truck to start. I heard the familiar cranking from the doghouse, then the whine of the powerful Mack engine as the truck came to life.

I pressed a different button, one next to the start switch. This was my only communication with the driver of the ladder truck. One ring meant STOP immediately, two rings meant go forward, three was for backing up. The tiller man rang first, letting the driver know all systems were go. The driver would respond with a like number of rings and the truck would roll. Two rings and Steve knew I was ready, he responded with two rings and we sped out the door. I slammed the bubble windows on the tiller cab shut which did little to keep the freezing December wind and chill from the inside. It didn't matter, though how cold or hot it was in the tiller cab, there was nowhere I would have rather have been. My turnout gear and the thrill of being a Providence Firefighter sitting on top of the world in a tiller cab were enough to keep me comfortable.

It takes a while to get the hang of the tiller, but once you do you never forget. It really isn't that hard, as one firefighter infamously stated, "any asshole can tiller," right before he crashed the tiller truck into the fire station.

The setting sun on the horizon offered little warmth on this cold winter's day; only the light when it disappeared would be missed, fleeting by the minute. The red and orange hues mixed with the grey winter sky as darkness seeped relentlessly through the brilliant colors, eventually replacing the beautiful canvas with black.

A mile away, two men frantically dug at the earth where their friend was buried alive. They were finishing up for the day when tragedy struck.

They were excavators, digging a foundation in a hilly embankment in the city's North End. The backhoe that they had been using sat idling at the crest of the enormous hole they had spent the day creating, never once considering it would become a tomb. The two men stood on the spot they last saw the victim before one of the walls collapsed, burying him under twelve feet of earth. They were afraid to use the machine that made the hole in fear of crushing or cutting their friend in half.

Once our crew had assembled we took over the rescue operation, sending firefighters into the hole in three man teams to dig. We set up emergency lighting, giving the scene the look of a movie set. This, however was no scripted story, this was real life, and sudden death. From inside the hole the silhouettes of firefighters holding tools resembling ancient weapons gave comfort to those digging. I trusted those shadows on the rise with my life should the earth shift and I become entombed.

We all had a turn. The ground was recently turned by the backhoe and easy to move. It was also potentially deadly. I looked at a twenty-foot wall of instability, waiting to crush us while I took my turn with the shovel, ever mindful of how fast a cave-in happens.

As the minutes pressed on the digging became more frantic. Eventually, Chief Moura had the backhoe operator carefully remove bigger mounds of earth, knowing every second was vital to the buried man's chance for survival. After taking a few scoops from the hole with the backhoe, our guys returned. My friend, Nate Sweet and two other firefighters were in the hole when we found the body. Just an arm, but the team was revitalized. The digging picked up steam as we tried desperately to free the man. Minutes flew by, oxygen was passed into the hole, and eventually a mask put on the man's face. We all watched as the three in the hole finally freed the victim, limp and lifeless from his grave. We placed him in a stokes basket and raised his body, passing him through us to safe ground. He never had a chance.

There was no transport, the medical examiner took over. We silently picked up our gear and went back to the station.

It was my first meeting with death. There would be many, many more. I've never gotten used to it.

It's different being with your friends and co-workers after living through a traumatic event. Strength in numbers comes to mind. Back at the station we talked about the incident while washing down the dirt covered shovels and portable lighting, feeling sympathy for the man who went to work that morning and never would come home, wondered if he left a wife or children. It makes it easier to share your thoughts with people who have lived through the same experience.

That was our last call of the day. We went our separate ways shortly after returning to the station. I had a half hour ride home. The incident was still with me all of the way. The emptiness of my car was suffocating; I couldn't wait to get home. Eventually I made it, looked at Cheryl, kissed her, hugged her and broke down. I don't think I cried for the man who died in the hole, I'm not even sure why I cried. All I know was it was good to be home and there was nowhere I would rather be.

Funny what runs through your mind when left on idle.

I park my car on the side of the building and let myself in. One shift to go. I don't feel like socializing so I sneak up the stairs into my office. The portable is on the desk, my leash, waiting for me to put it on my belt. It's going to have to wait a little longer.

I call fire alarm to tell them Rescue 1 is back in service then head to the shower. A good hot shower is equivalent to four hours sleep, and I can sure use some of that. The adrenaline rush from the stabbing is gone. I have one foot in the stall when the tone hits.

1847 hrs. (6:47 p.m.)

"Rescue 1 and Engine 10 a still alarm."

I must be tired. If I were thinking clearly I would have taken a shower then called fire alarm.

"Rescue 1 and Engine 10, respond to the corner of Niagara and Ontario for an MVA,"

"Rescue 1, responding."

Reluctantly I pull my dirty uniform over my tired and dirty body, grab my radio from the bathroom shelf and slide the pole. Mike is waiting, engine running and the same grin on his face that he started with last night.

"I called the chief and put in the paperwork. Your transfer has been cancelled, you have been permanently assigned to Rescue 1."

"Too late, this is my last shift, it's official," he says. We pull out of the station and head straight up Baker Street toward Broad.

I look over at him as he drives. I'm going to miss that goofy grinning, bald headed, fart machine. Well, maybe not the gas, I think and roll down the window.

"Right back at you," I say. He breathes deeply and basks in his deadly aroma.

Traffic is light so we keep the siren off during most of our response, only giving little squeals while driving through intersections. Engine 10 arrives on scene and gives their report.

"Engine 10 to fire alarm, inform rescue that we have an SUV wrapped around a utility pole, two ambulatory occupants possibly refusing treatment."

"Rescue 1, received."

"That's good, maybe we won't have to do anything," I say to Mike as we turn onto Ontario.

"Once they see the rescue they're going to see dollar signs. Guaranteed they suddenly have neck and back pain."

"Who are they going to sue, the utility pole?" I ask.

"They'll find a way," he says as we arrive on scene.

A black Jeep Cherokee has crashed into a pole, steam comes from the engine compartment. A crowd gathers; this is better than TV. I get out of the rescue and survey the damage, looking into the passenger compartment to see if there are any victims inside. Dan, Engine 10's officer, greets me.

"The guys over there say they're all set. People on the scene said they were the only two people in the truck."

"How do they look?" I ask.

"One of the guys looks a little dazed, the other one looks alright. The air bags didn't deploy so they couldn't have hit it that hard. You might want to get them to sign a refusal."

"I'll get it. Thanks."

Mike is talking to the occupants and has the story when I get there.

"These guys were driving to their friend's house when the steering wheel locked up. The driver says he tried to stop but couldn't so he swerved into the pole instead of going into the intersection. He's a hero!"

"If the steering wheel locked up, how did he swerve into the pole?" I ask Mike. It seems a simple enough question but the guys from the car appear mystified by it.

"I ain't going to no hospital," says one of them.

"Me neither," echoes the other.

They are wearing the uniform - baggy jeans, white sports jerseys and expensive sneakers. One of them has a Yankees hat tilted on his head.

"You don't have to go anywhere," I tell them. "If you are feeling any pain later you should go and get checked out. Sometimes it takes a while to feel any injuries."

"I don't have insurance," one of the guys says. The other nods his head.

They probably don't need medical attention but I wanted to give them the opportunity to refuse treatment. I get their names, put them on the state report with a brief description of the accident and document their refusal.

"I need you to sign this form. All it is is proof that you refused treatment," I say to them.

"I ain't signin nothin."

"Me neither."

They cross their arms and glare at me, as though I put the pole in front of them then drove their vehicle into it. One of them spits, just missing my foot, the other continues to glare.

Why me? These must be the biggest morons to ever walk the face of the earth. I have had enough.

"Quit being douche bags and sign the report!"

That woke them up. Lessons learned from Wayne have stuck with me when interacting in the inner city. Just because I'm a big dumb white guy from the suburbs doesn't mean I have to act like one.

They sign. I thank them and walk back to the truck, waving to Engine 10 as they pull away from the scene, headed back to the Broad Street Station and steaks on the grill. A police cruiser arrives, I give him the rundown and head back to the rescue, refusals in hand.

"Your people skills are remarkable," says Mike.

"Years of practice."

This is the perfect opportunity to give myself a break. We're heading back to quarters where I plan on basking in a luxurious shower in a leisurely fashion. It is Saturday night in the city. Things could get out of hand and probably will. It's just a matter of time. I want to be presentable for whatever the night has in store.

Back at the station dinner is being prepared. Art brought in some T-bone steaks and has them on the grill; the aroma of smoke and cooking meat has permeated the station, making me forget my misery, at least for a little while. I finally get into the shower, my portable radio close in case I need it. I haven't gone back in service and don't plan on it until after I'm done, and I am not hurrying. The water is as hot as I can bear and I let the spray hit the back of my neck. I just stand there for a few minutes and let the water work it's magic as my body starts to relax. I've only got about twelve hours left before I go home but it seems like an eternity. The radio continues to send rescues into the city for different reasons, none of them dire emergencies. As the hours grind on the radio becomes background chatter. All I can do is block out the transmissions and try to relax. My mind and body is numb from the days of abuse I have put it through, the shower helps me become clean again. If I can get through the next half hour without a run, I'll breeze through the rest of the night clean, well fed and refreshed.

"All Hot!" blares from the PA system as I'm drying off. I quickly get dressed and head for the steaks. The T-bones look as good as the smell advertised, thick, juicy and seasoned just right. Huge baked potatoes with sour cream and chopped chives are on the table; steamed broccoli sits on the stove waiting for us to dig in. The other guys let me and Mike go first; they know our time is short. I make a plate, sit down and get ready to feast. The first bite is delicious.

"Engine 13 a still alarm with an out of town rescue."

The guys drop their forks and knives and head for the poles. I just sit and look at my meal and think of what could have been.

"Rescue 1 to fire alarm, we're available."

"Roger, Rescue 1, respond with the 13's to 1332 Broad Street, in the plaza for a possible heart."

"Rescue 1 responding."

We wrap the plates in foil before we respond, leaving them where the guys were sitting. Mike and I put ours in the oven to keep warm. We won't be back for a while, Engine 13 should return before the food gets cold.

EIGHTEEN

1929 hrs. (7:29 p.m.)

"Engine 13 to fire alarm, do you have a better location?"
"The caller stated there was a man in a restaurant at that location who appears to be having a heart attack."
"Engine 13, received, we'll look around."

"Rescue 1 on scene."

Engine 13 is at one end of the plaza. We take the other. The plaza consists of a thrift store, a liquor store, a nightclub and a Chinese take-out. The 13's are looking for the victim in the nightclub and we are in the thrift store. We exit at the same time, make visual contact and give the universal sign of nothing yet by holding our arms upright and shrugging shoulders.

I find our victim in the Chinese take-out; a middle aged man unconscious, his face planted in an order of fried rice and General Tao's Chicken.

"Rescue 1 to fire alarm, the victim has been located in the restaurant."

"Engine 13, received."

We approach the man not knowing what to expect. I don't think he had a heart attack; this looks more like a seizure, alcohol intoxication or a diabetic emergency. Mike lifts his head from his dinner and I look into his eyes. Through the rice and oyster sauce I can see that they are glazed over and unseeing. I shake him gently.

"Buddy, what's going on?" I ask. He makes no reply and doesn't move. His pulse is strong and his respirations are regular.

"What do you think?" asks Mike.

"I don't know, maybe a diabetic. I'll try to find out what happened. Why don't you and the 13's get him in the truck and try to figure things out?"

"Right away," says Mike as the Captain, Steve, Jay and Art enter the place. Art and Steve have retrieved the stretcher from the rescue and are helping Mike load the patient onto it. He gives no help or resistance as he allows the guys to lift him onto the gig and wheel him out

"What happened here?" I ask the people behind the counter. They shrug their shoulders, claiming to have not seen a thing. There are three other people in the restaurant that I hadn't noticed until now. A mother and her two daughters are sitting at a table off to the side. The mom looks confused and her girls look scared. They are just kids, about eight and ten years old and have probably already seen too much.

"Did you guys see what happened?" I ask them.

"We were in line when he started shaking like he was crazy," said the older child. "He fell, then got back up, sat in his chair and fell into his food. My sister was crying and my mom didn't know what to do. Somebody called 911 then left." The other girl is gently sobbing while their mom talks to them in Spanish, probably trying to comfort them I surmise, listening to the soothing sound of her voice. The mom looks like a teenaged girl. Her children are wearing colorful dresses and new shoes with colorful ribbons in their hair. All three have luxurious dark hair and beautiful, soft dark skin. Easter Sunday is tomorrow, they look ready for the celebration.

"Tu edis baya," I say to them and they giggle a little. I think I told them that they look beautiful, but Renato, my Spanish tutor and with a little luck my new partner, once Mike leaves has an evil sense of humor and I may have said I smell like a monkey.

The patient is on the stretcher on his way to the rescue. I'm sure Mike and the guys have things well under control. I have a few minutes to help these kids. I sit on a chair next to them and let them know what happened.

"What you saw is called a seizure. A lot of people have them and they're not that bad, he is going to be fine when we get him to the hospital. He needs medicine and he will be as good as new. I'm sure that what you saw was pretty scary, but don't worry, you have been a big help. Without you, I never would have known what happened. Thank you very much for helping."

The kids are beaming from the compliments. It amazes me how such small acts of recognition go so far. I'm glad I stopped and talked to them. I'm not sure how it is that the kids speak English and their mom doesn't. There are a lot of undocumented immigrants in Providence. Often a woman will get to America and have a baby as soon as possible. The common term for these kids is "Anchor Babies." They are citizens of the United States of America as long as they are born on American soil. I see the desperate conditions these folks live in and can only imagine how bad things are where they came from. What I see is extreme poverty with a few luxuries, they must see things differently considering where they came from.

"Bye, now and thanks again," I say as they wave and I get in the rescue and shut the door.

Inside the rescue, Mike has the patient lying on the stretcher. He is still out of it but appears stable.

"You guys are all set," I say to Captain Healy. He would do whatever necessary if I asked, but there really isn't much more that they can do. The Thirteens head back to the station, and their dinner.

"He's postictal, blood pressure 140/100 and his pulse is 130," says Mike, giving his report while getting the IV ready.

"I wonder why his heart rate is so high?" I get the leads and put them on. His heart rate is fast, but without any other irregularities.

"Hey buddy, how are you feeling?" I ask him. He has come around a little, but is still confused from the seizure. He groans in pain.

"Dolor?" I ask.

"Si."

"Donde?" My Sesame Street Spanish will have to do, Renato only taught me how to flirt with women.

He points to his left leg. He may have injured it when he fell. Mike is already assessing the situation.

"Come se yama?"

"Jesus." He is coming around a little more.

"Jesus is right! Look at this!" Mike has cut the man's left pant leg and has exposed the bottom half of his limb. The smell coming from a gangrenous wound there fills the back of the rescue. I quickly open the side door and turn on the vents. Jesus has a festering sore that covers half of his shin and calf. Green pus and clear liquid is oozing through a filthy bandage and onto the stretcher. I cannot believe his condition. I will be shocked if the doctors can save the leg.

"What is his temperature?" I ask Mike.

"Wait a second." He gets the thermometer from its compartment, presses the on button, puts the end into Jesus's ear and waits for the result.

"One hundred and four! This guy is septic."

"Let's start a line and get him in." Mike gets going on the IV and I try to get more information. I have pretty much exhausted my Spanish vocabulary so this is difficult. I get an identification card from him and find out full name and address, which I copy onto the state report. Jesus has been living in misery for a long time from the look of his leg. He probably has no insurance and is possibly in the country illegally, which is probably why he has delayed seeking medical treatment. His decision may cost a lot more than deportation. Maybe where he comes from is a worse place than where he is and a leg is an equal tradeoff. I certainly wouldn't want to be forced to make that decision.

Mike has the IV line running and goes in front to drive. A few minutes later we are back at the ER.

Jan and Jim are working triage. The pace is frantic, three rescues are ahead of us and the waiting room is full. I wait my turn in the doorway; Jesus is sleeping on the hospital's stretcher that Mike and I have moved him onto. When I make it to the front of the line Jim is waiting.

"Hi, Jim, How are you?" I ask.

"Glorious."

I love it when Jim is working with Jan. They compliment each other perfectly, both voracious readers and freakishly witty. At times I try to match wits with them but find myself out-matched. They run triage better than anybody, the patients moved along in a professional manner, never missing a thing. People who are good at what they do are able to do their jobs with such ease that they are easily taken for granted.

"What have you got?" Jim asks.

"Fifty year old male, possible seizure at a restaurant, no trauma but he was witnessed falling from his seat onto a tile floor. Heart rate 130. BP normal, temperature 104. He's complaining of pain to his left leg and here is why." I take the towel covering Jesus's leg off. The smell hits Jim first. He shakes his head in dismay.

"Trauma," says Jim and leads the way. We wheel our patient through the triage area into the back where a medical team is assembling. Jim signs my report and takes over, explaining to the team the situation. The wound speaks for itself.

Mike is in the truck waiting for me.

"Are you still hungry?" I ask him.

"Starving," he responds. "Let's eat."

NINETEEN

The guys from Engine 13 have finished with dinner and are watching the Red Sox game. Mike and I find our leftovers where we left them. The radiant heat from the oven has turned my steak from a medium-rare masterpiece into a well-done piece of shoe leather. My drink is warm so I open the freezer for an ice cube or two and see the most beautiful thing I have ever seen. Sitting there, nestled between the empty ice cube tray and some frozen mozzarella sticks is a white cardboard box wrapped in a red ribbon. Not sure if I am dreaming I gingerly take the box out of the freezer and put it onto the kitchen counter. The ribbon is tied in a bow so I pull one of the loose ends and it falls from the box. Unable to take the suspense I open the lid. Two dozen manicotti lie inside in perfect rows. I have surely died and gone to heaven.

"Get your fat fingers out of the box," says Captain Healy as he walks into the kitchen. "Those are for lunch next week."

"I need them." It is all I can say, for the first time in my life I am nearly speechless. My good fortune is unbelievable.

"We're doing a Haz Mat drill Thursday morning so we picked those up when we got the ravioli. If you take them make sure you replace them."

"I'll replace them and I'll even buy lunch. I was supposed to pick some up for Easter dinner at my house but never made it. I can't believe these were in the freezer all week and I didn't know it," I say.

I take the keys to my car from on top of my desk and put them inside the box with the manicotti. There is no way I can leave the building without them.

"Did you know that those were in there?" I ask Mike.

"Of course."

"Why didn't you tell me?"

"You didn't ask."

My steak tastes better now that the saga of the manicotti is behind me. Sometimes things have a weird way of working out. The Red Sox have taken an early lead and I've showered and had a decent meal. The miracle of the manicotti has helped lighten my mood as well. I think my last ten hours might be bearable. The couch in my office is calling; it's time for a little snooze before the fun begins.

2049 hrs. (8:49 p.m.)

"Rescue 1 a still alarm."

I didn't even get a chance to sit down.

"Rescue 1, respond to 160 Broad Street for a man experiencing back pain."

"Rescue 1, responding."

160 Broad is home to Crossroads. The organization running the place used to be called Traveler's Aid and was founded years ago to help people who were from out of town and needed a place

to stay. They also provided comfort for weary travelers, directions and a cup of coffee. Their goodwill has metamorphosed from the intentions they were founded for into a homeless shelter. The people that benefit from the services provided there come from all walks of life. Most are good people down on their luck. They accept the help being offered until they can get back on their feet, then move on. For others, the agency and others like it provide a way of life that doesn't include productive achievement. The subculture that exists out of sight of every day citizens thrives in places like these. It is actually a lot of work figuring out where all the freebies are and how to get them. If the recipients of the handouts put as much time into working as opposed to figuring out ways to beat the system we would all benefit.

Providence's rescues are called to the "drop in center" at Crossroads numerous times every day. Most of our responses involve drug or alcohol abuse. Rhode Island Hospital is less than a mile from their location yet we are constantly being called there for non-emergency reasons. It is our job to help those in need, but we are constantly being called upon to help those who refuse to help themselves. In some ways we are acting as enablers to the people who refuse to be productive members of society.

We make it to Crossroads in four minutes. Standing outside is a man in his forties dressed in old jeans, sneakers and a hooded sweatshirt. Mike pulls the truck next to the curb where the man is standing. I unroll my window.

"Did you call for a rescue?" I ask him. He walks over to me with his hand on the small of his back and groans in pain.

"I have to go to Roger Williams," he says.

"Why?" Roger Williams is a privately run hospital about six miles from Crossroads.

"I've been moving refrigerators all day. I can't move, the pain is so bad."

I get out of the truck and stand next to the man.

"We'll take you to Rhode Island," I tell him.

"I can't go there, all of my doctors are at Roger Williams."

"What are their names?"

"Doctor."

That was a pretty good answer but there is no way I'm taking this guy across town to his hospital of choice when Rhode Island Hospital is a few blocks away.

"If you want to go to Roger Williams, take a bus."

"What are you busting my balls for? It's your job to take me, now let's go and quit fucking around."

Mike has joined me on the side of the truck.

"What's going on over here?" he asks.

"This jack-off wants to go to Roger Williams. He tells me it's my job to take him there."

"Fuck him." Says Mike, but in a nice way.

"Fuck you guys. This is unbelievable. I didn't want to do this, but you give me no choice. I'm a State Police detective. Now let's get out of here before you blow my cover."

"If you are a State Police Detective, I'm Osama Bin Laden," I say.

"Look, I'm a millionaire. I'll hook you up when we get to Roger Williams."

"You've got a deal. Let's go," I say.

Mike gives me a weird look as I help the nut into the rescue.

"Where are we going?" he asks.

"Rhode Island." I answer, out of earshot of the millionaire.

"I'm glad you finally caught on, they don't do anything at Rhode Island. At least at Roger Williams I'll get some medicine," he says.

"What kind of medicine?" I ask.

"Painkillers, what do you think."

I get his name, date of birth and all of the other pertinent information in the minute that it takes to get to the hospital. As soon as the back up alarms go off he is on to me.

"You took me to Rhode Island!" he says, shocked.

"What did you expect, a free taxi ride? You're lucky I took you anywhere. Get out."

He is pissed, but accepts his fate. The fact that three of the ER's security guards are outside the truck watching may have something to do with it. Elliot, Steve and Amir help me escort our "patient" in. I doubt he will be much trouble.

"What fabulous member of society are you gracing us with now?" asks Jim as he prepares his report.

"Forty-eight year old male, complaining of back pain since today as a result of moving refrigerators, originally demanded transport to Roger Williams because all of his doctors are there. He is alert and oriented, visions of his own grandiosity may be impairing his quest for potent painkillers."

"Glorious," says Jim and signs my report.

TWENTY

"That guy is nuts," says Mike.

"I don't know who's crazier, him or us," I say.

Things at the station are quiet. All I'm thinking about is getting some rest. An hour of sleep is what I need to get through the rest of the night. The reflection I see in the mirror while brushing my teeth is not pretty. Bags have developed under my eyes. No matter how many hour-long naps or ten-minute showers I get, the drawn and haunted look on my face will remain until I get some real rest. The hours are starting to take their toll. I don't think I'll be able to keep up this pace for much longer; it takes too long to recuperate.

Working in the same station as the engine and ladder companies is difficult. The temptation to hang up my rescue shoes and go back to fighting fires is sometimes overwhelming. The rescues are out running around like nuts, taking a beating day in and day out. The fire companies work at a more realistic pace. This job is not designed for us to constantly be on the move. Rather than being "on call," we are usually "on calls." Dealing with a constant torrent of other people's emergencies has a tendency to make one put their own well being aside. Before you know it some difficult life problems creep up on you and you find yourself ill equipped to deal with it. It's amazing how people in our profession can be so good at handling other people's problems, but so bad at handling our own. Numerous studies show that the divorce rate of people in the emergency services occupation is well above the norm. I happen to know the reason for that. You have to come through with the manicotti. It's that simple.

Every week I put myself through the same torment. In the end I always come to the same conclusion; I actually enjoy this work. I'm sure I'll feel refreshed and have a better outlook when I return next week after my days off. For now, I just have to quit being a bitch and suck it up. I call home. Cheryl picks up on the first ring.

"Hello."

"Hey, Babe, how's things?"

"Good here, how about you?"

"Can't complain."

"Yes you can and usually do."

"I know but I promise, no more complaining. The people just keep calling and calling. They never let up. If it weren't for all the nitwits this would be a piece of cake. The last guy we had was a real piece of work. He actually wanted us to take him across the city to Roger Williams so he could get more painkillers. I'm sure Darryl will be calling any second, he's due. The clubs will be getting out and you know how those assholes are, and I guarantee if they don't call some moron will crash his car or beat up his wife. If we don't get more rescues soon, I'm quitting."

"I'm glad that you're not going to complain anymore."

"Complaining never got me anywhere so what's the use? Anyway, Happy Easter. Do you need anything?"

"Everything is all set. The house is clean, Danielle is picking up my mother and Brittany is taking her home. I've got the ham seasoned with Heinz 57 and cloves, the veggies are ready and my mom is making the potato croquets."

"Excellent. I'm bringing the manicotti. Who's bringing the pie?"

"Tara made one and Dylan brought it over. We're playing cards with Bob and Tara on Monday.

"I hope they've been saving their money, I feel lucky."

"The way you've been playing you need to be lucky."

"Rescue 1 a still alarm."

2142 hrs. (9:42 p.m.)

"Rescue 1 respond to 96 Gallatin Street for a twenty-nine year old female complaining of abdominal pain."

"Rescue 1, responding."

"Got to go," I say to Cheryl.

"Be careful."

"I will. I'll see you tomorrow. Try to get to bed early and get some sleep."

"You too," she says.

"Love you, bye."

"Love you too. Goodnight."

For the first time all week, I get to the truck before Mike. A few seconds after I get in, he opens the driver's side door and sees me.

"An Easter miracle, you're here before me."

"The old guy still has some get up and go, you know," I say.

"My get up and go got up and went," he says.

"I hear you." Got up and went. Nice. Another one bites the dust.

Gallatin Street runs between Broad and Elmwood. Broad Street is starting to get busy again, the nightclubs are opening and the early crowd is coming in. The people on the street barely notice us as we pass. The drivers we share the road with are in no hurry to get out of our way. Mike changes the tone of the siren from the usual long wail to a series of chirps. That wakes up the guy in front of us who wouldn't get out of the way - he pulls to the side of the road.

We have to park in the middle of Gallatin, there are three cars parked in front of the house we are called to. I get out of the truck and walk through a gate in a chain link fence, up six or seven cement steps to a landing then knock on the door.

"She's in here," says a man who looks like a leftover roadie from 1980's Monsters of Rock tour.

"Why did you call?" I ask.

"She needs to get to the hospital," he answers, sounding more annoyed than concerned.

The patient is lying on a small couch in her pajamas. A small trash pail is on the floor in front of the couch. She leans over and vomits into it, then puts it down and lies back down. A lit cigarette burns in an ashtray near the pail of vomit. She is a big woman, at least two-fifty. Her hair is long, greasy and tied in a ponytail. The tip of the cigarette glows in the dim and smoky light as she takes a healthy puff. She rewards us with her exhaled smoke.

"How long have you been feeling sick?" I ask.

"Not that long. I had my liver replaced two years ago. An hour ago I had some wieners and a couple of beers and have been feeling sick since then."

"It doesn't sound like you need to go to the hospital."

"She's going," says her husband.

"Why don't you take her?" I ask.

"She'll get in faster if you do it," he says.

"You've got to be kidding me." I say.

The patient vomits again then starts gasping for breath.

"I can't breath!" she says. They win.

"Get your shoes and a coat, we'll take you," I tell her.

"I can't walk," she says.

"We are not carrying you. If you want to go to the hospital, get some shoes and your coat and let's go. Otherwise forget it."

"You guys had better carry her, she's sick," says the biker.

"I'll get the chair," says Mike. "It's easier than arguing and I want to get out of here."

I'm so tired that I go along with Mike. I just don't have the energy to get into a pissing contest with these people. The woman starts to vomit again. While she has her head in the bucket and Mike is getting the stair chair from the back of the truck I ask the guy the usual questions.

"What is her name?"

"Rose Wallace."

"Date of birth?"

"I don't know."

"She's your wife and you don't know her birthday?"

"What of it?"

"I think it's weird."

"Too bad."

Mike comes back and sets the chair up next to the couch. I ask Rose if she has the energy to get onto the chair. Slowly she makes the move, groaning and complaining the entire time. Mike rolls the chair to the door, and then I get a grip on the handles at the foot of the chair and lift. She weighs a ton, but Mike and I handle it without a problem. Mike rolls her to the rear of the truck where we transfer her to the stretcher then put her in the back of the truck. Her husband stands at the door and glares. We get in and close the door without him saying a word. No goodbye, no thanks, no nothing.

"What an asshole," I say to Mike once we are in back.

"I'll say," he responds. Rose neither agrees nor disagrees; she sits on the stretcher and looks miserable.

"120/80, pulse 90. Do you need anything else?" Mike asks.

"No, let's go. Rhode Island."

Mike gets out of the back, then into the front and starts the four-minute ride to Rhode Island Hospital. Rose moans and groans the entire way there, but thankfully doesn't vomit. I sit in my seat and watch the world go by. Mike is cranking Van Halen. Panama drifts from the cab into the back of the rescue, joining Rose, myself and the smell of stale cigarettes and vomit.

A young woman falls to her untimely death from an escalator in a shopping mall. Her bereaved family finds some solace knowing that her vital organs were put to good use, saving the lives of people in desperate need of them. It takes everything I have not to grab this patient by the throat and let her know exactly how lucky she is to be alive. I want to look her in the eyes, maybe squeeze her neck a little, and tell her just how lucky she is, and just how unlucky somebody else is that is dead, and what a waste she is making not only of her life and the second chance she has been given, but to the memory and legacy of the person who donated their very life essence to her so that she could smoke, drink, and eat "hot wieners" to obesity. Instead, I sit behind her in the Captains seat and fill out the report, leaving my commentary to myself.

Triage is packed with sick, injured and drunk people. Jan is still at the desk and greets us as we wheel Rose in.

"What have you got?" she asks.

"Twenty-nine year old female, liver transplant two years ago, vomiting for an hour possibly related to some hot wieners and beer she had a while ago."

"Why did she eat hot wieners?"

"Good question."

Jan signs the report. We hang around the hospital for a while, but none of our rescues are there, and Jan and Jim seem bored with us so we head back to quarters.

The radio chatter drones on. Rescue 2 is on Friendship Street for an assault, Rescue 3 was sent to help a twelve year old with emotional problems, Rescue 4 is headed to Thayer Street for an intoxicated female and Rescue 5 is transporting thirty-six year old male who "smoked too much crack," and wants his heart checked.

"I've got a big day planned, I hope we get some rest," says Mike.

"Me too. Too bad all of the rescues are out. I don't think we'll even make it back to the station," I say.

"Maybe we'll have another Easter miracle," says Mike.

"We can only hope."

I've spent a lot of time on rescue yet I never stop hoping for a quiet night. I've never had one, but the old timers tell stories of the days when people called the fire department only for emergencies. Legend has it that long ago people only called if somebody was really sick or hurt. I wish we could go back to those simpler times, but I know it will never happen. There is a culture, mostly located in the bigger cities that are dependent on government services. We have allowed this way of life to fester, and until our leaders smarten up, the problem will get worse. The "what can you do for me" attitude is spreading and until a major policy shake-up occurs, will continue to grow. Providence doesn't need more rescues; more people need to take responsibility for themselves and stop looking for a free ride.

"See you in the morning," I say to Mike as we make our way upstairs.

"Sleep tight. Don't let the bedbugs bite," he says as the door to his dorm closes. I laugh to myself, lie on the bunk and slip peacefully into unconsciousness.

TWENTY-ONE

0015 hrs. (12:15 p.m)

"Rescue 1 a still alarm."

"Rescue 1 and Engine 10; respond to 1844 Broad Street for a reported shooting, stage for the police."

Bedbugs shoot.

"Rescue 1, Responding.

"Happy Easter," says Mike when I get to the rescue. The door goes up, Rescue 1 goes out, the door closes. A popular nightclub is located at 1844 Broad Street. Numerous violent incidents have occurred here over the years. The City Council passes an ordinance every now and then in response to the latest debacle, the business is closed for a while, only to re-open a few weeks or months later under a different name. The latest incarnation has been doing a great business for about a year without incident. Apparently all of that has changed.

"Engine 10 to fire alarm, police on scene waving us in."

"Rescue 1, received."

A large crowd has gathered in front of the nightclub. The people making up the mob move as one from my vantage point through the windshield, about four blocks ahead. The flashing lights from Engine 10 and the dozen or so police cars give the illusion of a strobe light and a late night fog has descended on the area, giving the scene a movie set quality. The crowd parts as we approach, the mood almost festive. Two or three fist-fights have started on the fringes, the emotions high. The "scene is safe" and we follow the lights from Engine 10 toward the victim. He is lying on his side in the gutter, unconscious, three bullet holes in him, one in his shoulder, another his left hand and the one that worries me most, the right side of his abdomen. At least there was no head shot.

I still find it amazing the ability inherent in some people to point a gun at another human being, aim, and pull the trigger. These are not crimes of passion or revenge, rather just idiotic drunken bar fights gone out of control because the kids in the 'hood are "packing." Instead of a nice, old-fashioned fist-fight, maybe a broken nose and some bruised knuckles the next day, these arguments are settled with gunfire. I can see from the excitement in the faces around me, as we push the stretcher through the crowd, that this is something these kids will talk about for months.

"I was there," will be heard on the streets as word of the shooting spreads. The witnesses and participants will get instant "street cred" just for being there.

The guys from Engine 10 help us get the victim on the stretcher and roll him into the rescue. We don't encounter much resistance from the crowd, but that is not always the case.

Closing time on the weekends is a raucous time in Providence. Some of our rescue crews will go downtown and park near the clubs and enjoy the sights while waiting for the inevitable call to come in. Ryan and Ray were working Rescue 1 last year on a typical Friday night at closing time. They went to the famous Haven Brothers Diner for a late night snack and parked near one of the clubs and waited for a call. The call came to them instead.

A crowd was leaving one of the bars. Before long the Rescue was surrounded by people. As Ray and Ryan sat in the truck, a man pulled a gun, twenty feet in front of them, pointed it at another man and shot him, point blank range numerous times in the head. He died instantly and dropped to the ground. More guns were drawn, Ryan radioed for Police and Ray attempted to back out of the area until the scene was secured. The angry crowd had other plans for the rescue. The truck was blocked in, Ray and Ryan forced to administer assistance at gunpoint. The crowd was all black guys, Ryan and Ray caucasian. A tentative racial truce exists during normal daily routines, what rears its ugly head in times of duress is horrible. I have felt the rage from minorities during similar situations and it is truly frightening. Anything can happen when emotions spill over and rules of tolerance, acceptance and racial diversity are interrupted by violence. The fact that the violence has nothing to do with two white guys sitting in a rescue watching one black man blow another black man's head off is irrelevant and lost when the mob reacts to violence.

We got in and closed the doors. Dan was in charge of Engine 10 and knew how things worked in these situations. I was able to concentrate on the patient, Dan got Paul to drive the rescue, gave me Keith in back and cleared the path. We worked while rolling toward Rhode Island Hospital, Engine 10 leading the way through the mob.

"I need vitals, an EKG, and an IV, I'll get the 02. Cut the clothes."

Mike had the trauma shears and was busy cutting through the dying man's clothing, Keith put the blood pressure cuff around the man's right arm and I took a non-rebreather from the overhead compartment, filled the reservoir and put it in place.

"80/40, pulse 138," said Keith, now working on the EKG leads. Mike had done as good a job as he could with the guy's clothing, most of his body was now exposed. I didn't see any more holes. I fished through the remnants of his jeans looking for an ID and found one in his back pocket, no wallet just a state issued ID card. I have no idea if this is actually my patient, it could be his older brother, cousin, or an imaginary person who is of drinking age. Mike nails the IV on the first shot. I pick up the phone and hit the preset number for the Triage desk at Rhode Island. Melanie answers after three rings.

"Providence Rescue 1, I've got a twenty year old male, unconscious, hypotensive and tachycardic gunshot wound to his lower abdomen, shoulder and hand, IV established, 02 going we'll be there in a minute."

"See you when you get here," says Melanie. I know that she is now calling for a Level 1 A Trauma Team. Doctors, Trauma Nurses, Respitory, ER Techs and the blood bank are assembling in one of the trauma rooms waiting our arrival. The fact that this kid got shot within three miles of the area's best and most experienced trauma teams is in his favor. His chance of survival is slim, but he will have a fighting chance thanks to the people about to take over his care. The folks in the rescue happen to be the best around as well, which is another plus.

Paul backs the rescue in and we wheel our patient past a number of EMT's and patients from surrounding communities and into trauma alley. Melanie meets us and leads us to Trauma Room 3 where the team awaits. Because of the expert help in back of the rescue, I've had time to assemble the story, patient's condition and treatment thus far and relay it to the waiting trauma team. They don't want to hear any opinions, treatment suggestions or other commentary, nor should they. They are waiting for the facts. I let them have them.

"Twentyish year old male found in gutter, unconscious, gunshot wounds to his left shoulder, left hand and lower left anterior quadrant, hypotensive at 80/40, elevated heart rate at 140, unconscious during EMS response, 16 gauge IV established left AC, 02 enroute, pulsox 100% during transport EKG shows sinus tack." While I relay the information the patient is moved from our stretcher to theirs. We put him on a backboard and applied a cervical collar on the scene which helped immobilize him during transport and now makes moving him easier. Another reason is if CPR become necessary a hard surface is necessary. I hope it doesn't get to that point.

We have done all we could, I back out of the trauma room and let them do their thing. Our response was quick, transport minimal and treatment almost immediate. Time is everything in these situations and we did our part in extending this kid's life. It's up to him now, and surviving the ER will be just the beginning of his battle.

The ER resembles Grand Central Station at rush hour, rescues coming and going, sick people, injured people, drunk, lonely people, all looking for a cure.

TWENTY-TWO

0144 hrs. (1:44 a.m.)

"Rescue 1 and Engine 10, a still alarm."

At first I'm not sure if the shooting was a dream. I remember Mike telling me we were done for the night, sitting at my desk to catch up on reports then lying on my bunk. Now, the fluorescents are blinding me and the noise from the PA system making me deaf. I sit up and put my feet on the floor. The joints are the first things to go. Sharp pain shoots up my legs from my knees. My back joins the chorus as I try to stand upright. My elbows and neck creak and groan as I hobble to the stairs. I'm afraid if I slide the pole I might forget to hold on and crash to the floor. I must resemble a Neanderthal man leaving his cave.

"Rescue 1, respond with Engine 10 to the corner of Thurbers and Prarie for an MVA."

"Rescue 1 responding."

Engine 10 is first on scene and reports one victim with neck and back pain. We arrive a minute later to find the patient sitting in the driver's seat of a mini-van holding the back of his neck and groaning in pain. A small car is a foot behind the mini-van. Neither vehicle has any visible damage.

"The driver of the car says he barely touched the bumper," says Dan from Engine 10.

Mike checks on the injured party and I talk to the driver of the other car. He speaks no English, but through an interpreter who witnessed the "accident," I learn that the collision happened at about two MPH when the guy in the mini-van stopped short and the other guy tapped him from behind. The other driver isn't hurt so I join the other guys at the mini-van.

"Let's get it over with," I say. Mike has already gotten the long backboard and a cervical collar from the rescue and is applying it to the patient. The guys from Engine 10 help extricate him from the van, pulling him out of the vehicle, while laying him on the board and putting him onto the stretcher. The van will be towed to a local service station. The police arrive on scene as we are pulling away with the patient. The officer will have to go meet the patient at the hospital to finish his report.

"Where is your pain?" I ask my patient as we drive toward Rhode Island Hospital. Mike has assessed the patient and finds that his vitals are stable.

The man speaks limited English and I speak extremely limited Spanish, but between us we get the information we need. The hospital is still cranking. The relentless stream of patients that the hospital treats is amazing. Melanie is back at her post, handling things with amazing grace. You would never know that a short while ago we left her with a patient full of holes and clinging to life. She manages to make everybody feel as though they are the only patient in the world, be they gunshot victims, drunken college kids or barely injured motor vehicle accident victims. Somehow, she manages to make angry, exhausted rescue guys feel like they are the only people in the world as well.

We leave our patient on our backboard where he will probably stay for a long time. Non-critical patients are seen in the order in which they come. If his back wasn't hurt before, it will be after lying flat for a few hours. I am not proud of the fact that this gives me a great deal of morbid satisfaction. There is a chance that the patient really is hurt, and we did everything that we are required to do while extricating and transporting him.

I'm thankful that my shift is almost over. I'm losing my perspective. The driver of the other car is caught up in a scenario that plays over and over, all over the country. The ugly "Make them Pay!" monster has reared its ugly head. The guy lying in the hospital may get a little money, but the real victim is the poor slob who tapped an opportunistic faker. His auto insurance will increase, possibly to more than he can afford putting him in the position of not driving or breaking the law and going without. The only people to benefit from this unfortunate incident are the lawyers.

I help Mike put the truck back together so it will be ready for the next emergency. We pass a Cranston rescue as we make our way out of the parking lot and back to quarters. The bar crowd is out. Hopefully they will make it home safely. As annoying as they are, I would rather respond to a thousand fake calls than one real one where somebody gets killed.

TWENTY-THREE

Every minute of rest is imperative at this hour. It is simply not natural to be on alert for thirty-four hours.

0305 hrs (3:05 a.m.)

"Rescue 1 and Engine 13 a still alarm."

My mind takes a few seconds to realize that we're heading out again. The rest of my body will have to catch up. I get up again, knowing that the despair I'm feeling will dissipate as the minutes go on. At this hour I usually go from anger when the tone hits to despair when I get to my feet, to acceptance by the time I get in the rescue to anticipation while en-route. When the anger refuses to make way for the rest of the emotions it's time to get off the truck.

"Rescue 1 and Engine 13, respond to 26 Jillson Street for a diabetic."

I get to the bottom of the stairs and realize I've forgotten my portable radio. Shit. Back up the steps. Engine 13 roars out of the station, Mike waits with the engine running and lights on. At the top of the stairs he hits the siren, thinking I must have slept through the alarm. I haven't missed a call yet, no reason to start now. I retrieve the radio from the charger next to my bunk, turn around walk back into the hallway and slide the pole, landing at the rear of Rescue 1.

"What's the hold-up?" asks Mike, grinning again.

"You're going to look awfully funny with that siren up your ass," I say.

"Promises, promises," he laughs and we're on our way to Jillson Street.

"Engine 13 to Fire Alarm, advise Rescue 1 we have a fifty-five year old male, diaphoretic and unconscious, assessing vitals."

"Rescue 1, received the message." I put the mic back in the cradle.

"I bet he doesn't even know what diaphoretic means," I say to Mike.

"He probably wouldn't know a blood pressure from a blood vessel."

"He probably never even felt a pulse."

"He probably doesn't even have a pulse."

"That's because he doesn't have a heart."

"He has a heart it's just a tiny little thing the size of an appendix."

"How big is an appendix?"

"As big as Captain Healy's heart."

"Rescue 1, on scene."

Captain Healy meets us at the door.

"You're gonna need the stair chair, he's out cold."

Mike has already retrieved the chair from the rear compartment, I've got the blue bag. There are a few steps before we enter the home, a small entryway, then a straight run of stairs to the second floor. We get up the stairs and find our patient, soaked from sweat, lying in the middle of a king sized bed, dressed in a sleeveless t-shirt and pajama bottoms. A woman, who I assume to be his wife, is standing next to the bed holding a glass of orange juice.

"Do you know his glucose level?" I ask her.

"We took it at eight it was 110."

"Is he insulin dependant?"

He takes it morning and night.

Mike has straddled the bed to get a more current blood glucose reading.

"Twenty-two, he hit the jackpot!" he says, raising the glucometer in the air like a trophy. He has a way about him that enables him to be his usual crazy self without upsetting patient's family members. People can usually see when a person is genuinely decent, even if they do act a little weird.

Arthur has the IV kit open and is fishing around for the necessary equipment. Captain Healy has cleared a path for us, moving a dresser and a throw rug out of the way. Jay and Steve have joined Mike on the giant bed and are dragging the patient to the side. I put on some protective gloves and get to work.

I remember my first diabetic emergency. I was a firefighter assigned to Engine 2 when a call came in for an unconscious female. We responded to a beautiful home on the East Side and found a middle-aged woman face-down on her kitchen floor. Her seven-year-old granddaughter called 911 when she found her grandmother and couldn't wake her. The child was hysterical when we arrived, I had no idea what was going on. Kenny Loux, the driver of Engine 2 that day, had about three years experience then and had seen a number of similar situations. He made sure the woman's airway was clear, listened for breath sounds then checked her pulse. The rest of us kept the little girl calm and waited for the rescue. These were the days before Fire Companies were equipped with automatic defibrillators, IV equipment and medications. All we could do was CPR, administer oxygen and wait for a rescue. Luckily, no CPR was necessary on this day. Kenny said that he thought this was a diabetic but he wasn't sure, it could be an overdose, heart attack or any number of things.

After what seemed an eternity, Rescue 5 arrived on scene. Lieutenant Dave Raymond walked into the room and immediately went to work. I watched as he opened the blue bag, started an IV, drew up some medication and delivered it, all while explaining things to the woman's granddaughter. Thirty seconds after the medicine entered her bloodstream, the woman on the floor's eyes twitched. Then she moaned. Then her eyes opened. She sat up, looked around and asked, "what happened?" Dave calmly told her that her blood glucose dropped and he had to give her an amp of D-50 to get her back. She looked around her, saw all of the firefighters but was only concerned for one person in the room; her granddaughter. The girl ran to her then, hugged and kissed her, clung on and wouldn't let go.

I thought I had witnessed a miracle. I'm not 100% sure but there is a very good chance that I decided on that day to eventually transfer to the rescue division. It took ten years, but here I am.

Arthur hands me the IV equipment then opens the box of D-50. I apply a tourniquet to the patients arm and search for a vein. Diabetics can be hard sticks, and Milton is no different. I want to use a large bore needle to better administer the D-50, which has the consistency of maple syrup, but from the look of things a twenty-gauge catheter will have to do. A couple of pats on the inside of the elbow and I think I see a vein. I rub some alcohol over the site and drive the needle home. Bingo, first shot, the little reservoir at the end on the catheter fills with blood letting me know I'm in. Mike takes over, fastens the drip set and adjusts the flow. Arthur pushed the D-50 through the IV line and into Milton's bloodstream.

It is quiet. We're all standing around the bed, waiting. First the eyes flutter, and then open. Milton looks around, sees six firefighters in his bedroom with his wife, shakes his head and says, "sugar went low."

"Very low, you were in insulin shock," I say.

Prolonged insulin shock can result in permanent brain injury. Milton probably took his insulin then neglected to eat properly. Overexertion can also be a cause. Whatever the cause, this was a serious medical problem.

"We're going to take you to the hospital," I say as Mike gets the stair chair ready.

"I'm not going to no hospital."

"Yes you are," I say, not very convincingly, I'm afraid.

"Thank you boys for helping, but I ain't going, and that's that."

"You have to go, what if you're your sugar drops again."

He's drinking the glass of orange juice and his wife has some peanut butter and crackers on the bedside. I'm reasonably certain that he will be fine, but I would much rather take him in for an evaluation.

"He won't go," says his wife.

"This is a serious situation," says the Captain. "You really should go to the hospital. Think about your wife, what would she do if something happened to you?"

That almost cracked old Milton but he is a stubborn guy. He's not going, and that is that.

Mike hands me a refusal form. While I fill out the necessary information, the guys clean up our mess and file out of the bedroom. Milton signs the refusal.

"Good night folks, and good luck," I say as Mrs. Milton shuts the door behind me. I'll have to find a way to replace the D-50 we used getting Milton back to the world of the living, but I'll let Vinny worry about that, he'll be here in a couple of hours.

Engine 13 leaves a cloud of exhaust as they pull away from the house on Jillson, Mike and I get into the rescue and close the doors in time to avoid the toxic cloud.

I consider forgetting to go back in service but pick up the mike instead.

"Rescue 1 in service, signed refusal against medical advice."

TWENTY-FOUR

0415 hrs (4:15 a.m.)

We back into the station. The tone hits. The overhead door closes, then rises.

"Rescue 1, Engine 11, Ladder 5, Special Hazards and Battalion 2, respond to 367 Reservoir Avenue for a reported tipover."

"Rescue 1 on the way," I say into the mike as we head out the door. A few minutes later Engine 11 comes over the radio and transmits their findings.

"Engine 11 to fire alarm, inform all companies we have a confirmed tipover, we'll keep you informed."

When there is a report of a tipover, which means a vehicle is on its side, or a rollover, which means a vehicle has gone completely over, a rescue, an engine, a ladder, Special Hazards and a chief officer are dispatched. Any number of things could go wrong, or already have on these calls, and the more manpower on scene, the better chance of helping the victims.

I put some protective gloves on as we close in. I hope nobody is hurt too badly. Ladder 5 and Battalion 2 arrive on scene at the same time we do. I can still hear the siren from Special Hazards wailing in the distance; they had the longest trip to the incident. Joe, the officer of Engine 11 has had time to investigate. He gets on the radio and gives an update.

"Engine 11, inform all companies that the vehicle is empty, we're looking for victims."

As we arrive on scene, I look around the immediate vicinity but don't see anybody. If the occupants were thrown from the car their chances of survival diminish. The Hazards arrive and join the rest of us. We take a good look around the area and surmise that whoever crashed the car has managed to walk away. The car is resting on the passenger side and sits up against a utility pole. There is major damage to the vehicle. The person or persons in the car are lucky to have not been killed. This could be a stolen vehicle. Another possible scenario is a drunk driver cracked the car up then managed get out of the car and will call report the car stolen later. A worse possibility is the person involved has a head injury, or had a diabetic emergency prior to the crash and is wandering around somewhere critically injured. All of the companies who responded will keep their eyes open on their way back to their stations. Joe gets back on the radio.

"Engine 11 to fire alarm, put all companies back in service, victims have fled the scene. Inform police of the situation."

Upon returning to the rescue I get a surprise. Doc, the officer in charge of Special Hazards is waiting there for me. I've been on the job for a long time, Doc twice as long. We have crossed paths numerous times. Up until this point in my career he has never said a word to me. I don't think he has even looked in my direction. He has a reputation as a great firefighter and a no-nonsense officer but a terrible cook. It was my understanding that he views the rescue division with contempt, and the rescue officers more so. He looks right at me as I walk toward him.

"Are you the guy that wrote that article?" he asks.

"Uh, yea," I respond like a moron.

Doc looks me in the eye and extends his hand. I take it and we shake.

"That was great," he says, and then walks back to his truck.

"What was that all about?" asks Mike as I get in.

"You wouldn't believe me if I told you," I say.

Doc's compliment means a lot to me. I'm glad I wrote that article. I wish I hadn't misjudged Doc.

"Engine 11 and Rescue 1 a still alarm."

"Here we go again," I say to Mike. We wait with Engine 11 to hear where we'll be going and watch the other trucks head back to quarters. The night is moving along. I have less than four hours before my relief comes in.

TWENTY-FIVE

0435 hrs. (4:35 a.m.)

"Rescue 1 and Engine 11, respond on Route 95 North, right before the Thurbers Avenue curve, for an MVA."

"Rescue 1, responding."

We leave the scene of the tipover and head to the wreck on the highway. There are only a couple of other cars on the road now. We ride behind Engine 11 and get onto 95 headed north to look for the accident. Sometimes the caller gives the wrong information. Sure enough, we pass an accident in the high-speed lane of 95 south. It appears to be a two-car crash.

"Rescue 1 to fire alarm, there is an accident on 95 southbound in the high speed lane right after the Thurbers Avenue curve. We'll keep you advised if there is anything on 95 North.

"Roger, Rescue 1. Engine 11 receive?"

"Engine 11, received the message. There's nothing ahead of us, we're turning around and heading south."

We follow Engine 11 as they take the next off ramp, then onto the next on ramp and head back to the accident scene. The damage to the vehicles didn't look too serious as we passed in the northbound lanes, but you never know what to expect until you get up close. Engine 11 pulls behind the wreck to provide protection and we pull in front.

The first vehicle appears empty and undamaged. The other one has major drivers side and front end damage. Three people are in the car. I approach on the passenger side and look into the passenger compartment. Two young women are in the rear seat helping the driver; both have blood up to their elbows. The driver is a semi-conscious man who is around the same age as the girls. The side window is smashed, air bags have deployed and there is deformity to the steering wheel. One of the girls is holding a blood soaked rag against the left side of the man's head.

"We're going to get you out of here," I say to the people involved as I look into the passenger side window. I know the driver needs help but I don't know about the other two.

"Are you two okay?" I ask.

"We're fine, but he's lost a lot of blood. We were behind him when his car went out of control. He spun around, then hit the Jersey barrier."

"Thanks, but what about you two?" I want to know if an additional rescue will be needed.

"We weren't involved, we just stopped to help," says the girl holding onto the guy's head. I look at them and see concern on their pretty, blood and tear streaked faces.

"Do you know him?" I ask.

"No, but he needed help. We're nursing students at Rhode Island College."

This is just what I need about now. All week I've been helping people. Some have desperately needed it, others haven't. The driver of the demolished car needed help and two people were good enough to give it. He was lucky. The best most of us do is call 911 from our cell phones and drive away, letting somebody else handle the bloody mess. What these girls did may not be the smartest or safest thing to do, but it is the most courageous. My faith in humanity is restored.

"I didn't think anybody cared," I say.

Mike and the crew from Engine 11 have the stretcher and backboard ready. Mike nudges me out of the way and puts a trauma dressing on the man's head then wraps it with a roll of cling wrap. The blood soaks the dressings and immediately starts dripping down his face.

"I think he has an arterial bleed," says Mike.

"Let's get him out of here."

I get out of the way and let the firefighters do their thing. Rick and Cindy from Engine 11 have the man extricated, collared and in the rescue in about a minute. His head still bleeds profusely. I give a bottle of peroxide, some sterile water and a few towels to the nursing students. It's the best we can do. I hope they never lose the humanity they have just shown. Years of taking care of other people takes its toll, but some people are able to hold onto their compassion.

"Blood pressure 98/60, pulse 120," says Mike. I get an oxygen mask ready and Cindy starts an IV.

"Do you need a driver?" asks Joe, from Engine 11.

"As soon as we get the IV started." I say.

Rick gets in the drivers seat; Cindy and Mike stay in the back with me.

"All set, head to Rhode Island," I say to Rick after Cindy establishes IV access. The truck moves, slowly at first, then picks up speed. The patient is saying he's sorry over and over.

"What is your name?" I ask.

"Patrick. I'm sorry," he answers.

"Do you remember what happened?"

"I'm sorry. I was driving and I lost control. I'm sorry, I might have been going too fast."

"What is your date of birth?" I ask, while simultaneously transcribing the answers onto the State report - no easy task in the back of a rescue speeding down route 95.

"I'm sorry. Twelve, twenty, eighty," he answers.

"Do you have any medical problems?"

"I'm sorry, what do you mean?"

"Asthma, diabetes, cancer, anything like that." I say.

"No, but I have ADD."

"Do you take any medications?"

"Adderol. I'm sorry."

"You don't have to be sorry. You had an accident, they happen all the time."

"Yeah, but I've been drinking."

"Well, nobody but you got hurt, maybe the State Police will give you a break." I say.

"They have to. I'm in the criminal law program at Roger Williams. I want to be a cop. I've ruined everything now."

"Maybe not, like I said you might catch a break."

"I'm sorry. Can I call my mom? She just got a divorce. She doesn't need to worry when I don't come home."

"We'll call from the hospital. Try to relax, things will work out."

I hope things work out for him. One small mistake can ruin a person's life. Instead of a future with the police department, this poor kid might be working at a department store. I have a tendency to look at drunk drivers like they are the biggest assholes on the face of the earth. I conveniently forget my own dubious drunk driving exploits. I am lucky I was never caught. The self-righteous bullshit I sometimes throw at the drunks I pick up is just that; bullshit. Very easily I could be in their shoes, and I am not alone. Thankfully, I smartened up before I made a costly mistake. With the help of Bill W. and millions of other recovering alcoholics, I managed to put my life back together, one day at a time.

The rescue backs into the bay at Rhode Island Hospital. What a surprise, it's almost five in the morning and there are three Providence rescues and four from other towns there with us. The back doors open and Rick starts to pull the stretcher out. I've slowed the IV to a drip, barely enough the keep the vein open. Too much IV fluid is contraindicated in head injuries. We wheel Patrick through the doors, past the waiting rescue crews and their patients and to the triage desk. Melanie takes a look at the patient. I give her a brief description of what happened and she decides to put him into a trauma room because of the arterial bleed.

"Can you call my mother?" he asks again.

"What's the number?" I ask. He tells me and I write it on the report.

Back in the rescue, I pick the cell phone up and call the kid's mom. She answers on the first ring. After a few tense moments, I convince her that Patrick is alive and well.

I know how it feels to wait and worry for missing children. My two have always made it home, sometimes later than they were supposed to, but they always made it. I cannot imagine the grief that comes from losing a child. The most heart-wrenching image from my career to this point is that of a mother and father walking down trauma alley toward their dying son. He fell from a seven-story building onto a concrete driveway. He was a college kid sneaking onto the roof of his dormitory for a smoke after a stressful exam week. It was something he and his friends did all the time.

This time though, he slipped on the icy shingles, falling eighty feet. His friend watched him go over the edge and frantically called 911 from his cell phone. I found a crumbled mess at the foot of the building. We did what we could. The boy's name was John. He was conscious while we rushed him to the trauma room at Rhode Island Hospital. He tried to communicate with us, but his ruined body wouldn't allow it. He grabbed me with his broken bones and looked at me through eyes that had been dislodged from their sockets as we rode to the hospital. We were supposed to be his rescuers, but we knew, and I think he did too that he didn't have a chance. That ride was the longest five minutes of my life.

He was alive when we got him to the trauma room. His parents were notified and began their forty-five minute journey to their son's side. I was sitting on the floor in the corridor of trauma alley, finishing my report when they arrived. The look of hope mingled with horror and fear was etched on their faces as they made the long walk to the end of the hall. His mother clung to her husband as they walked; he held her up and carried her. I am thankful that I wasn't in the room when they saw the mangled body of their son. He died the next day, his parents by his side.

Light has entered the world; darkness begins its morning retreat. The birds that have adopted the awning above the rescue bay announce the start of a new day with their joyous chirping. Sunrise is still hours away, but a new day begins to form. All I want to do is go to bed. One look at Mike in the driver's seat tells me that he feels the same. Patrick will be fine. Unfortunately, not everybody is as fortunate.

TWENTY-SIX

The station is quiet when we return. I think our work is done.
The city seems at peace. My bunk is calling me. Unfortunately, so
are the citizens of Providence.

"Rescue 1 a still alarm."
*"Rescue 1, respond to 1 Washington Avenue for an intoxicated
student."*
"Rescue 1, on the way."

Mike drives toward the intoxicated student while I doze in
the passenger seat. We ride for a few minutes, and then arrive on
scene. Once there we are escorted by security through the lobby of
the dorm toward one of the rooms on the second floor. We have
brought the stretcher and fit it into the elevator.

The halls are empty, except for a security guard and us. The
smell of alcohol permeates the space. The aroma must be seeping
from the pores of the student body, as this is a dry campus. The
kids do their share of partying on the streets and in the clubs of
Providence. Our victim is face down on a bunk in one of the tiny

dorm rooms. I try to wake him but he is out cold. No other students are around.

We have been through this countless times. Mike turns him on his side and gets hold of his belt. I cradle his head and lift his upper torso in tandem with Mike. We drop him onto the stretcher. Mike has an ammonia cap and puts it under the patient's nose.

"What are you doing?" I ask.

"Waking him up," he responds.

"What are you doing that for?"

"So you have somebody to talk to on the way to the hospital," he says.

The kid shakes his head back and forth when the ammonia hits his brain. He comes around a little, and then slips back into unconsciousness. I'm glad. I hope he sleeps all the way to the Emergency Room.

We wheel him out of the dorm and into the fresh air. The morning chill revives him a little, but not for long. We put him into the truck and head toward Rhode Island Hospital. On the way I take his vital signs and find they are normal for a drunken kid his age.

Melanie is gone. The day shift has taken over the ER.

"What are you doing working on Easter?" I ask Katey as we wheel our patient in.

"The same thing as you," she says, and then adds, "Go home, you look awful."

She signs the report. I'm done. Mike has the truck running and takes off as soon as I sit down.

I can see the sun crack the horizon between the giant fuel tanks that line the shore. A tanker slowly makes its way down the Providence River to dock at one of the tank farms. I guess we're not the only ones working on Easter Sunday. I can't see it, but I feel Providence's skyline looming behind us as we quietly travel Allens Avenue toward the station.

Vinny has just pulled his car onto the ramp. He is the same age as me, but looks much younger. Mike puts the flashing lights on and backs us into the station. I get out of the officer's seat and hand the radio over to Vinny. The torch has been passed once again.

EPILOGUE

He must have been sleeping; the phone rang for a long time before he picked it up.

"Hello."

"Nado, it's me, are you sleeping."

"Not any more."

"Sorry to wake you up but this is important. Do you remember that sick girl we had this morning?"

"The one from PC?"

"Yeah, her. The chief just called me. Turns out she had bacterial meningitis and we were exposed. They want us to report to Roger Williams immediately for treatment."

"Wow, it she all right?"

"They read her last rights, it doesn't look good."

"Shit."

"I know. Want us to come by and get you, I'm working overtime, Rescue 6."

"Nah, I'll drive, it's right around the corner."

"All right, see you there."

Rescue 6 was added to our miniscule fleet of Advanced Life Support vehicles about a year ago. It hasn't helped us out much, just kept the surrounding communities at bay for a little while.

They still come to Providence on mutual aid in disproportionate numbers.

I snapped my phone closed and sat back in my chair, closed my eyes and let the news sink in. Earlier in the day we had responded to Providence College for a "student vomiting". It was Tuesday morning, the day after a three-day weekend. I'd have bet the rescue that this was a call for a kid with a hangover. It took about five minutes to make the trip from the Allens Avenue Fire Station to the Providence College Campus. Renato was at the wheel as he had been for the last couple of years, filling in for Mike who left the rescue division for a spot on Engine 15 in the Mount Pleasant section of the city. I still see Mike occasionally on calls, at least he stayed on the same platoon. He's the same, always on, always making me laugh no matter how miserable I might be.

Ladder 3 had been dispatched along with Rescue 1 and gave me their report as we turned into the campus.

"Ladder 3 to Fire Alarm, advise Rescue 6 we have a twenty year old female dizzy and disoriented, have them bring the stretcher."

"Rescue 1, received."

Most of the time the students are able to walk to the rescue. This kid must be pretty sick, I figured. I helped Renato get the stretcher from the back of the truck and walked toward the Health Center, located just below the dormitory where a student fell to his death a while ago. I pointed to the spot that he landed.

"That's where the kid fell," I said to Renato.

"I know," he said, probably tired of me telling him again but wise enough to not to remind me that I tell him the same story every time we come to PC. That is one of the many reasons I thank the Rescue Gods every day that he was transferred to Rescue 1 a few weeks after Mike left. Sometimes things have a way of working out.

She looked sick, but then so many of them do after a long weekend. Providence College has its fair share of parties. Inside the health center Ladder 3 finished taking vital signs. Nelson, a firefighter who came on the job years ago with me and still looks a lot like Wayne Newton gave me the story.

"She's 21, started throwing up last night at midnight. No medical history, doesn't take medications and has no allergies. She seems a little confused."

Usually our college aged patients walk to the rescue, not her. Her name was Kellie, her Irish name as beautiful as her face. She tried to answer my questions but her words were garbled. I became worried about her condition; we transported her immediately to Roger Williams Hospital. Renato drove in his usual way, I never felt a bump or turn in the road. En-route Kellie started to have some seizure-like activity. As she vomited I handed her a basin. She didn't understand what it was and threw up on herself instead. She shook as I held the basin to her face, and then fell back on the stretcher when I let her go. Her eyes couldn't focus on mine. I put her on a non-rebreather with high flow 02 and let her rest. I felt that her skin was cool and damp as I swept the hair from her eyes.

The nurse at the hospital took my report and immediately got her into a room where the Doctor on call saw her. I heard them mention a bleed as I washed the sweat and vomit from my hands. I had just taken off my gloves to do the report when she got sick. Five people were working on Kellie as I left. The Doctor said it is probably a head bleed from an injury or meningitis. Rather than a head bleed, I hoped it was meningitis and whatever got on me had been washed away.

The chief called at 2200 hrs and told me to report to Roger Williams Medical Center. Kellie had bacterial meningitis and we were exposed. I had hoped she didn't have a bleed in her brain but I never expected this. Viral meningitis is bad, but not deadly. Bacterial meningitis kills. It seems every year I read in the paper some poor kid who came to college and caught this bacterium somehow and died. Kellie's family was with her in the Intensive

Care Unit. She was intubated and fighting the infection, but was in critical condition. I had to wait until morning to see if she would live or die. As for me, I took a big dose of Cipro and let it work. The medicine made me sick, but not as bad as Kellie. I stayed on duty until the morning, poking my head into Kellie's room whenever I had the chance.

After a long couple of days I got word that Kellie might pull through. She had been extubated and woke up for a little while . She knew who she was and where she was but wasn't quite sure what had happened. She was lucky. Her roommates made her seek medical attention instead of going to sleep, which is what she wanted to do. The infection was caught before doing irreparable damage. Six firefighters and about forty staff and students were given antibiotics as a precaution. Her roommates saved her life. I love a happy ending and hoped things continued to improve.

As things turned out, things did improve. After multiple seizures and days of uncertainty, then weeks in bed, then months in therapy Kellie made a full recovery.

One day, months later I found an envelope addressed to me in the top drawer of my desk at Rescue 1. It was from Kellie's family, thanking me for my part in saving their daughter and sister's life. I must have read the note inside the card a hundred times, then a few more. This job has the strangest way of grabbing you by the throat when you least expect it. When I heard how sick Kellie actually was, after I had taken the mega dose of Cipro and was back at the station, alone in Rescue 6's office I had what I now call a mini-meltdown.

It is said that every critical incident we live through takes a little piece of our heart. We are able to keep all of the pieces stored somewhere, hoping to put everything back together some day. Kellie's incident took a bigger part of my heart than I realized. Maybe hers was the piece that was holding the rest together. I sat in the office that night, in between Cipro furnished runs to the bathroom and wondered, after all these years, if I was going to be able to hold on for many more. Maybe it was the memory of John falling eighty feet to his death from the roof above us when we carried Kellie out, maybe it was the knowledge of my own two girl's frail existence on this earth or maybe I had just had enough. Had she not pulled through I doubt if I would have stayed on the Rescue, I had just seen too much. While she fought for her life in a hospital room three miles from my location, I fought nausea, diarrhea and severe depression in a cramped temporary office at the Atwells Avenue Fire Station.

I can't say that I prayed to God or the rescue gods or even asked for any intervention at all; I will say that by night's end, I managed to sort things out enough to let it all go and let nature, or whatever, run its course.

I met Kellie and her family on her graduation day from Providence College. She's going to be a teacher.

She's off to a great start.

ACKNOWLEDGEMENTS

Many thanks are in order. Cheryl, Danielle and Brittany, who are the reason for everything I do. Jon Ford, confidante extraordinaire. The Men and Women of the Providence Fire Department, "In Omnia Paratus." Thank you all. Erin, bookseller extraordinaire. My friends from the Blogosphere, in the general order I found them, or they found me, Ambulance Driver, Chrysalis Angel, Happy Medic, Pink, Warm and Dry, Paramedic Supermonkey, The EMT Spot, TOTWTYTR, Burned Out Medic, A Power Within, Street Watch, Medic 999, Cabin Fever, I Just Call it as I See It, Life in Manch Vegas, The Brick, Ghetto Medic, Not Trained but we Try Hard, Notes From Mosquito Hill, Siren Voices, Pondering, The Insomniac's Guide to Ambulances, Unlimited Unscheduled Hours, Report on Conditions, Medic Dani, A Life in the Day of a Basic's Doc, Swordmaster's Apprentice , Everyday EMS Tips, and everybody from the Fire/EMS Blogs Community, as well as the dozens of other blogs I enjoy. Thank you for the great reads and inspiration.

ABOUT THE AUTHOR

Michael Morse lives in Warwick, RI with his wife, Cheryl, two Maine Coon cats, Lunabelle and Victoria Mae and Mr. Wilson, their dog. Daughters Danielle and Brittany live nearby. Michael spent twenty-three years working in Providence, (RI) as a firefighter/ EMT before retiring in 2013 as Captain, Rescue Co. 5. His books and articles offer fellow firefighter/EMT's and the general population alike a poignant glimpse into one person's journey through life, work and hope for the future.